The Healing Power of Meditation

The Healing Power of Meditation

Leading Experts on Buddhism, Psychology, and Medicine Explore the Health Benefits of Contemplative Practice

Edited by Andy Fraser

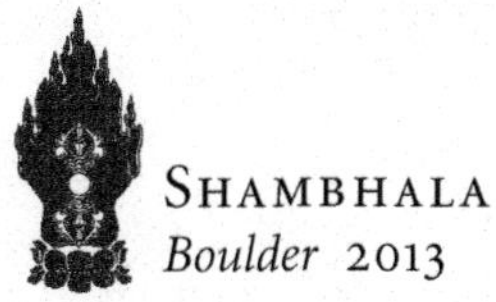

SHAMBHALA
Boulder 2013

Shambhala Publications, Inc.
4720 Walnut Street
Boulder, Colorado 80301
www.shambhala.com

Some parts of chapter 10, by Ursula Bates, originally appeared in Trish Bartley, *Mindfulness-Based Cognitive Therapy for Cancer: Gently Turning Towards* (Chichester, UK: Wiley-Blackwell, 2011), 289–302.

9 8 7 6 5 4 3

Printed in the United States of America

♾ This edition is printed on acid-free paper that meets the American National Standards Institute z39.48 Standard.
♻ Shambhala Publications makes every effort to print on recycled paper. For more information please visit www.shambhala.com.

Shambhala Publications is distributed worldwide by Penguin Random House, Inc., and its subsidiaries.

Library of Congress Cataloging-in-Publication Data

The healing power of meditation: leading experts on Buddhism, psychology, and medicine explore the health benefits of contemplative practice/edited by Andy Fraser.—First edition.
pages cm
Includes bibliographical references and index.
ISBN 978-1-61180-059-3 (pbk.: alk. paper)
1. Meditation—Therapeutic use. 2. Meditation—Buddhism. 3. Buddhism—Psychology. I. Fraser, Andy, 1973–
RC489.M43H43 2013
615.8'528—dc23
2012050297

Contents

PART THREE

Mindfulness in Health Care

PART FOUR

Meditation and Spiritual Care

Acknowledgments

Deepest thanks and appreciation go to the following people for helping to make this book a reality:

To all of the contributors for sharing their wisdom, expertise, and unique perspectives on the subject of meditation and health—and for their patience and assistance in preparing their chapters for publication.

To everyone at Rigpa International and Lerab Ling in France who was involved in organizing the conference that inspired this book, including Judith Soussans and Jan Linehan, Ally Cassidy, Céline Demarcq, Volker Dencks, Andy Fitzgibbon, Mylène Ghiglione, Eszter Hoffman, Anthony Morrey, Indira Rosenthal, Vinciane Rycroft, Sam Truscott, and Yessica Younes; and to Laurence Bibas and Olivier Raurich for facilitating the presentations.

To Patrick Gaffney, Philip Philippou, and Kimberly Poppe for their wise counsel, and all those who assisted with editing, translation, and transcribing, including Nancy Adess, François Audétat, Karien Bezemer, Simone Blatti, Helen Cargill, Tim Carstairs, Mary Deeks, Thomas Demarcq, Helen Depret, Linda Forrester, Phoebe Frame, Winie Froeling, Elizabeth Fukushima, Anahita Hamidi, Kathy Hammer, Ian Ives, Norman Jackson, Amy Jennings, Gela Krug, Karen Lane, Sylvie Marleau, Aline Maurer, Julie Milstien, Marian O'Dwyer, Paula Overgoor, Tineke Peeters, Julia Pruy, Sébastien Reggiany, Indira Rosenthal, Janet Savin, Isabella Schlenz, Linda Selis, Erric Solomon, Marlou van Hoorn, Marieke van Vugt, Christine Westlake, and Stephanie Wimmer-Davidson.

Foreword

by Daniel Goleman, PhD

In the mid-1970s in Cambridge, Massachusetts, some of the seeds were planted that would bear such splendid fruit four decades later at Lerab Ling, a meditation center in the south of France. At Harvard, Richard Davidson and I, with the help of Clifford Saron, were doing research on attention training and on meditation as an intervention in stress reactivity. In the mid-1970s these topics were not yet on the map of mainstream psychology, and our work was not received with much enthusiasm.

Nearby, a recent PhD from MIT, Jon Kabat-Zinn, was beginning his program in Mindfulness-Based Stress Reduction for patients with chronic medical conditions, a then-new approach to helping people manage long-term illnesses in a way that would improve their quality of life. His work, too, was greeted with skepticism. Yet we all shared an underlying conviction that these applications of contemplative practice had great validity and could be of benefit to many, if given a chance. Our certainty stemmed in large part from our own experiences in Buddhist practice. In those days empirical evidence was sparse.

Slowly, over the years, those convictions have been borne out by scientific findings that strongly support the notion that our states of mind have an impact on our health, and on how we relate to the body's inevitable failings. And meditation has proved to be one of the most powerful paths to managing our emotions in ways conducive to well-being.

We have come a long way since our early forays into this field, as the 2010 Meditation and Health congress at Lerab Ling attests. Like the conference itself, this book brings together leading experts from diverse backgrounds and specialties—Buddhism, neuroscience, and medicine—to explore from different angles how meditation can be most beneficial. Some of the major researchers in this area—Clifford Saron, Sara Lazar, Jon Kabat-Zinn, and Erika Rosenberg among them—report their remarkable findings. On the Buddhist side, Sogyal Rinpoche, whose vision came to fruition with this conference, and Khandro Rinpoche offer a traditional context and a foundation for these beneficial practices.

This book not only includes some of the latest scientific research and charts the history of how meditation became more mainstream but also offers much practical application. It features people explaining how they integrate meditation out in the world, sharing their experiences and advice, and gives moving examples of how meditation has touched people and brought widespread benefit. These stories are told in a fascinating variety of voices, hard to find elsewhere: Ursula Bates's work in hospice care, Edel Maex's and Lucio Bizzini's endeavors in psychiatry, Cathy Blanc's trainings for doctors and nurses, and Rosamund Oliver's teaching meditation to prison officers and caregivers. This range will be inspiring for health-care professionals—or anyone—who might be looking to introduce meditation in their work, or simply to try it for themselves.

I'm delighted to see that these proceedings are being shared with a wider audience in *The Healing Power of Meditation*. And I'm pleased to see that the subject is treated in an engaging, accessible way, rather than with the dryness of an academic journal. I truly hope this book will reach the widest possible audience, so that this good news can be received by many.

Introduction

A few years ago I had the opportunity to interview the Tibetan Buddhist teacher Yongey Mingyur Rinpoche. As he sat cross-legged in a big armchair, dressed in his red monk's robes, I asked him about his experiences as a guinea pig for scientific research into the effects of meditation. The results of this research had led to his being labeled "the happiest man in the world," and I was curious to find out exactly how this unassuming, softly spoken Tibetan lama had come to receive such an impressive title (which, as you might expect, he did not take particularly seriously).

Mingyur Rinpoche told me how, in 2002, he had been invited to the laboratory of the renowned neuroscientist Richard Davidson at the University of Wisconsin, Madison. Eight monks, each with between ten thousand and fifty thousand hours of meditation experience, were asked to perform a range of different meditation practices. As they did so, Dr. Davidson and his team employed cutting-edge brain-imaging equipment to measure exactly what was going on inside the monks' heads. Mingyur Rinpoche recalled how he had been instructed to lie on the retractable platform of an fMRI (functional magnetic resonance imaging) machine, which shows brain activity by detecting changes in blood flow. Once his head had been immobilized, earphones fitted, and a blanket draped over his robes to protect him from the cold, he was positioned inside what he described as a "big white coffin."

For another test, he was fitted with an EEG (electroencephalogram) recording net, which used 126 electrodes placed against his scalp to measure changes in electrical activity deep within his brain. When he began to meditate as instructed, something strange occurred. The machine malfunctioned. Or at least that is what the researchers thought had happened, because their instruments were telling them that the frequency of electrical signals in the subject's brain had increased to an alarming level. When they recalibrated the machine and started over, the same thing happened again. The gamma-band oscillations were the largest that had ever been recorded in humans, with the exception of people in the grip of extreme states such as seizures. Mingyur Rinpoche explained, "Normally, when the level of gamma waves gets to a certain point, you are totally crazy, out of control. They got these results from many other meditators too, not just me. When we meditated, the gamma waves increased above normal levels, and when we stopped meditating, the waves decreased."[1]

The data collected by the researchers in Wisconsin indicated that these Buddhist contemplatives, far from being crazy, were able to exercise a remarkable degree of control over their brain activity, generating mental states that were precise, focused, powerful, and lasting—even when loud noises that most of us would find extremely disturbing, such as a woman screaming or a baby's plaintive cries, were piped into their ears without warning. In short, the conclusion was that long-term meditation practice can change the structure of the brain, wiring into us a range of positive effects and tendencies, such as enhanced concentration levels, increased contentment and well-being, a greater capacity to cope when faced with challenging circumstances, and an ability to experience feelings of intense compassion that leave us primed to go to the aid of others.[2]

These results captured the public imagination, and photographs of monks being examined in the laboratory appeared in the pages of *Time* and *National Geographic.* The eye-catching images of robed Tibetans wearing EEG "hairnets" became a powerful symbol of the coming together of their ancient tradition with the investigative tools of modern science. The wave of research that had been instigated since the turn of the millennium at laboratories in Madison, San Francisco, Berkeley, Princeton, Harvard, Paris, and Zurich—and the results that were subsequently published in respected peer-reviewed journals—established the credibility of the emerging field of contemplative neuroscience. Meditative methods that had been developed and perfected over centuries in the East were standing up to serious scrutiny under lab conditions, and were being shown to have major implications for the mental and physical health of people in the modern world. Perhaps most significant, the science was also showing that these benefits were accessible to all; there was no need to spend half one's life sitting in meditation or to embrace any particular religious faith or ideology.[3]

A Pioneering Conference

This was the context in which a group of scientists, health-care professionals, and meditation teachers came together in 2010 for the groundbreaking conference on meditation and health that provides the content of this book. Over two days they presented some of the latest scientific and medical studies, shared Buddhist perspectives on meditation and the mind, and gave firsthand accounts of how meditation is being applied in health care today. It would not be an exaggeration to say that all of these remarkable individuals have, in different ways, been pioneers in the gradual process of bringing meditation into the mainstream, and offering its benefits to the widest possible cross-section of society. Each presentation has been made into a chapter of this book—edited, clarified by the speakers themselves, and, in some cases, updated to integrate the most recent research.

This book mirrors the conference itself by charting how meditation has developed from a New Age novelty into a powerful tool for alleviating suffering in the modern world; by sharing profound insights on meditation and the mind from the heart of the Tibetan Buddhist tradition; and by revealing some of the latest scientific evidence showing meditation's potential to benefit a wide range of people, in surprising ways.

The Meditation and Health conference was the third in a series of International Forums on Buddhism and Medicine (see www.buddhismandmedicine.org) that were initiated by the Tibetan Buddhist teacher Sogyal Rinpoche to discuss new approaches to treating and healing physical and mental suffering. The first, in 2002, was entitled Physical Pain and Suffering, while the second, in 2006, addressed the subject of Depression: Mental Suffering and Healing. The 2010 forum was the first major conference in Europe to explore in detail the health benefits of meditation, and it drew an audience of scientists, doctors, nurses, psychologists, psychotherapists, and other health-care professionals, as well as many interested members of the public. All were given the chance to experience different types of meditation for themselves, both during the presentations and in special sessions led by meditation instructors.

The conference took place in a rather unusual convention center: a traditional Tibetan temple located not in the lofty peaks of the Himalayas but in the beautiful countryside of Southern France. Frédéric Rosenfeld, a psychologist who opened the conference with a history of meditation and health over the past century, remarked that it was the first time he had delivered a presentation without wearing shoes! Yet it was entirely fitting that this temple should host such a gathering, for not long before, it had been inaugurated by one of the most vocal champions of Buddhism's increasingly fruitful interaction with the contemporary world, His Holiness the Dalai Lama.

Buddhist Perspectives

In his role as Tibet's spiritual leader, the Dalai Lama has encouraged pioneering teachers such as Sogyal Rinpoche and Jetsün Khandro Rinpoche (who both spoke at the conference) in their efforts to make the wisdom teachings of the Tibetan Buddhist tradition accessible and relevant to people today. Sogyal Rinpoche was among the first Tibetan teachers to travel and teach widely in the West, and over the past forty years he has introduced many thousands of people to meditation, either in person or through his best-selling book, *The Tibetan Book of Living and Dying*. He has founded meditation centers around the world, including the temple at Lerab Ling in France, and he has instituted programs to share the essence of the Buddha's teachings with health-care professionals, caregivers, and business leaders. In chapter 1 he presents a vision of meditation as a master key that enables us to understand, tame, and transform our mind, unlocking our potential for healing on the deepest level.

Like Sogyal Rinpoche, Khandro Rinpoche has skillfully managed to build a bridge between the Tibetan Buddhist tradition, which for centuries remained isolated from the rest of the planet, and the modern world. Having grown up in a Tibetan community in exile, she now holds joint responsibility for one of Tibet's most ancient and influential monasteries, which was reestablished in northern India by her father, Mindrolling Trichen Rinpoche. At the same time, her command of the English language and keen grasp of Western culture have enabled her to teach meditation and Buddhist philosophy to people of all backgrounds. In chapter 2 she challenges us to put aside all preconceptions about what meditation might be. Meditation has nothing to do with spirituality, she says. Rather, it is an invitation to examine and dismantle our habitual ways of looking at ourselves and the world around us: "The most important thing is that you are able to recognize this tremendous inner power and capacity that you are endowed with, and that you spend time with it."

Scientific Evidence

As well as supporting the authentic transmission and preservation of the Buddhist tradition, the Dalai Lama has made it his mission to promote the engagement of Buddhism with science, health care, and education. Much of the meditation research that is presented in this book very likely would not have been possible without his encouragement and the personal connections and networks that he has forged with the scientists involved. His childhood fascination with the workings of clocks, movie projectors, and cars as he was growing up in Tibet's capital, Lhasa, developed into something far more significant when the Dalai Lama began to engage in discussions with scientists such as David Bohm, Carl von Weizsäcker, Karl Popper, and Francisco Varela. He shrugged off skepticism from critics who argued that the two types of inquiry—contemplative and subjective on the one hand, scientific and empirical on the other—are fundamentally incompatible and that any attempt at collaboration would be a waste of time.

Since 1987 the Dalai Lama has hosted annual dialogues with leading psychologists, scientists, and philosophers, under the auspices of the Mind and Life Institute. It was at one of these meetings, in 2000, at the Dalai Lama's home in Dharamsala, India, that he initiated the flurry of research activity in which Mingyur Rinpoche and his fellow monks took part. "All of these discussions are very interesting," the Dalai Lama said, "but what can we really contribute to society?" The challenge was clear. The more scientists were able to examine, evaluate, and publicize the benefits of meditation, the greater its potential to help people would be.

More and more research is being undertaken, and papers are being published at an ever-increasing rate. As Frédéric Rosenfeld recounts in chapter 3, this association of meditation, science, and medicine has come a long way since the early attempts to study yoga practitioners in India in the 1920s. In 2007 the largest study on meditation to date was conducted in Colorado. The Shamatha Project is a multimillion-dollar venture involving sixty nonmonastic meditators, a handpicked team of researchers from around the world, and some of the most sophisticated scientific equipment and psychological assessment techniques available. In chapter 4 the lead scientist, Clifford Saron, presents a fascinating overview of the Shamatha Project and an analysis of its results so far.

Researchers such as Erika Rosenberg and Sara Lazar belong to a new generation of scientists who are dedicating their careers to investigating the effects of meditation on the brain and the emotions. In chapter 5 Rosenberg gives a scientific view of how emotions work. She explains why they have such a powerful influence on our lives, how meditation can help us to intervene at each stage of the emotional process, and what the resulting benefits are for our mental and physical health. In chapter 6 Lazar presents some of her most recent research on the effects of meditation on the brain. Using an MRI (magnetic resonance imaging) scanner, she has shown that meditation can bring about structural changes in parts of the brain that are important for processing emotions, as well as a decrease in the size of the brain's "fear center."

Part two reflects the core mission of this book: to investigate, evaluate, and present the benefits of meditation. The scientists themselves are far too professional to draw sweeping conclusions about the implications of their work. Many of these areas of inquiry require further investigation, they insist, and the results must be duplicated. An editor can be more cavalier, so I attempt to summarize some key findings of these studies. You can decide for yourself, as you hear from the scientists in their own words, whether I have exceeded my brief.

Meditation increases our well-being, mindfulness, empathy, resilience, and ability to handle our emotions. It decreases depression, anxiety, and neuroticism. More specifically:

- Meditation reduces activity in the amygdala, a part of the brain associated with fear and anxiety, and causes the amygdala to become smaller.
- Meditation protects the brain's cortex from the effects of aging and can boost the production of telomerase, an enzyme that plays a crucial role in protecting cells from premature aging and has been linked to longevity.
- Meditation increases our ability to perform tasks that involve perceiving small visual differences, and to maintain focus for long periods of time.
- Meditation increases activity in parts of the brain that have

been linked to depression, anxiety disorders, schizophrenia, and bipolar disorder.

- Meditators who showed increased levels of mindfulness were also found to have lower levels of the hormone cortisol, which is linked to stress and can adversely affect physical health.
- Meditation brings about structural changes in regions of the brain that are important for emotion regulation, empathy, and self-referential processing. Intensive meditators show increased engagement and sympathy when they see others suffering.[4]

Meditation and Health Care

Scientific research would, of course, be merely a fascinating and expensive distraction if its discoveries had no practical use beyond the confines of the laboratory. It is significant, therefore, that in recent years institutes have been established at several leading universities in the United States with the specific purpose of examining how meditation, as well as practices related to the cultivation of compassion, can be applied in the wider world. This is of particular relevance in fields that require a high level of emotional intelligence, such as education, health and social care, and business leadership.

One of the most powerful examples of this movement of meditation into the mainstream has been the success of mindfulness. Mindfulness had its humble beginnings in the basement of the University of Massachusetts Medical School. It was 1979, and a young PhD in molecular biology who was also a meditator, Jon Kabat-Zinn, had become convinced that basic meditation techniques could help people who were "falling through the cracks of the health-care system." Presenting a few fundamental meditation methods in a simple, structured, and secular way, Kabat-Zinn developed an eight-week program that he called Mindfulness-Based Stress Reduction (MBSR). He persuaded physicians to send him patients who had failed to respond to more conventional forms of treatment, and as the patients started to show results, the referrals kept coming. Although Kabat-Zinn's patients were telling him that mindfulness worked, his training as a molecular biologist had taught him the importance of an evidence-based approach. He responded by instigating a number of pioneering studies on the health benefits of meditation, particularly for the treatment of chronic pain, stress, and anxiety. (Kabat-Zinn provides a detailed account of his work in chapter 7.)

Fast-forward three decades, and millions of dollars are being spent each year on research into the clinical applications of mindfulness, with much of that funding coming from the National Institutes of Health. Mindfulness-based programs have sprung up all over the world, including Mindfulness-Based Cognitive Therapy, which has been remarkably effective in the treatment of recurring depression. Kabat-Zinn has introduced meditation to cancer patients, drug addicts, prisoners, lawyers, businessmen, and combat veterans, to name just a few. I once heard a professor of psychology observe, "If these techniques were a pill, they would create a megabucks market."

Starting with Jon Kabat-Zinn himself, we hear in parts three and four from health-care professionals in the United States, the United Kingdom, France, Ireland, Switzerland, and Belgium who have been inspired by their personal experience to bring meditation or mindfulness practice into their work and share it with their patients. Along the way all of these medical practitioners have experienced awkward moments—from Kabat-Zinn's sleepless night before presenting his Mindfulness-Based Stress Reduction program to the Dalai Lama to Rosamund Oliver's encountering skeptical looks on the faces of staff at one of London's most notorious jails when she arrived to teach them how to meditate. Always, their response was to find ways to present the benefits of meditation in simple, straightforward language and to back up their explanations with published research. Often they left the word *meditation,* with all its cultural and religious baggage, out of the initial conversation entirely. Their stories paint a vivid picture of the challenges involved in this groundbreaking work, and the rewards that it can bring when people discover meditation for the first time.

The psychiatrist Edel Maex begins chapter 8 with a guided meditation. Mindfulness, he explains, is all about how we relate to our thoughts, feelings, and emotions. When we find a "middle way" between suppressing them and being carried away by them, healing becomes possible. This is of particular significance for those who suffer from depression, where negative thoughts can run riot and spiral out of control. In chapter 9 Lucio Bizzini gives a detailed outline of the Mindfulness-Based Cognitive Therapy program that was developed specifically as a treatment for depression. To complete our section on mindfulness, Ursula Bates describes the delicate process of working with palliative-care patients at a hospice in Ireland. As she explains in chapter 10, many of her patients encounter mindfulness when they are at their most vulnerable, both physically and emotionally. As they engage with the practice in the final weeks or months of their lives, the consequences can be extremely profound and powerful.

Spiritual Care

In addition to mindfulness-based programs, there have been many other initiatives to share meditation with people from all backgrounds. Rosamund Oliver and Cathy Blanc were pioneers in a field that is now known as spiritual care, sometimes called contemplative care. With the guidance and support of Sogyal Rinpoche, who introduced them to meditation, they have developed ways to share specific practices from the Tibetan Buddhist tradition with people in positions of care or responsibility, such as doctors and nurses. The pressures on those who have a duty of care can often put them under great personal strain, leading to compassion fatigue and burnout. In chapter 11 Cathy Blanc describes how she took on the daunting task of bringing these methods into hospitals and clinics in France, where the separation between church and state is strictly observed. In our final chapter, Rosamund Oliver details her efforts to teach meditation in institutions such as jails and hospices, where, despite her initial reservations, she found the staff to be extremely receptive to learning meditation.

Once a symbol of the counterculture, *meditation* is now a household word, routinely discussed in the media, used by the advertising industry to promote all kinds of products and lifestyle choices, and practiced in its various forms—both spiritual and secular—by millions of people. Ask the contributors to this book where they think all of this will lead, and they describe a not-too-distant future in which meditation is practiced in schools, hospitals, retirement homes, hospices, offices, jails, and households around the world, not in the name of any particular religion or belief system but simply because it is good for us. To paraphrase Khandro Rinpoche, if the day does come when we are all walking around with abnormally high levels of gamma waves suffusing our brains, looking like contestants for World's Happiest Person, then the Buddha himself—the one who put meditation on the map 2,500 years ago—would no doubt be very happy indeed.

ANDY FRASER
January 2013

PART ONE

Buddhist Perspectives on Meditation and Health

1

Understanding the Mind and Meditation

A Buddhist Approach to Well-Being

Sogyal Rinpoche

Sogyal Rinpoche is a world-renowned Buddhist teacher and the author of The Tibetan Book of Living and Dying. *In this chapter he explains that the essence of the Buddha's teachings, and our most important task in life, is to understand and transform our mind. It is meditation that helps the mind to settle, unlocking its extraordinary power of healing and bringing us a deep sense of stability, contentment, and well-being.*

Regardless of who we are, the main purpose of our life is to be happy. You could call it the heart of being human, because we all share the same wish, and the same right, to seek happiness and be free from suffering. But then if you take a closer look, you can see that there are two kinds of happiness. One is based more on physical comfort or pleasure and is the happiness of the senses, whereas the other is founded on a deeper kind of mental contentment. The former can be very expensive and also turn out to be quite unsatisfying, whereas the latter will not only bring you complete satisfaction but also doesn't cost a thing.

Many people these days spend lots of time and energy trying to accumulate material things. This means that they have little or no chance to think about developing inner qualities such as compassion, understanding, patience, and contentment. So when they are faced with the difficulties and stresses of life, they find it very hard to cope. Yet a person who is in touch with that deeper sense of contentment and inner peace will find that his or her mind can still be happy and at ease, even when going through serious crises and suffering. This explains how some people can have every material advantage and yet still remain discontented, while others are always satisfied and content, even living amid the most challenging of circumstances.

The great Buddhist saints of the past used to say that only the foolish look for happiness outside of themselves. The wise and the learned, they say, know that happiness and the causes of happiness are all already present and complete within us. This is why His Holiness the Dalai Lama often points out that the principal characteristics of genuine happiness are inner peace and contentment. Have them as your basis, he advises, and your mind will be relaxed and at ease. And if your mind is relaxed and at ease, then no matter what difficulties or challenges you encounter, you will not be disturbed and upset, because your fundamental sense of well-being will not be undermined. You will be able to carry out your everyday tasks, your work, and your responsibilities more efficiently, and you will have the wisdom to discern what to do and what not to do. In turn, your life will become happier, and when problems do occur, you will even be able to turn them to your advantage.

Once our minds are more at peace, both inner and outer harmony automatically follow. As medical and scientific research continues to show, our mental states, and the ways in which we deal with stress and emotions, have an enormous impact on our physical health and overall well-being. What could not be clearer is how crucially important it is that we take care of our minds.

Understanding the Mind

The entire teaching of the Buddha can be summed up in a single line: "To tame this mind of ours." In other words, "To tame, transform, and conquer this mind of ours." The great masters often say that this one line captures the essence of the Buddha's teachings, because, if we can understand the true nature of our mind, this is actually the whole point—of both the teachings and our whole existence.

The Buddha himself said that all fear and anxiety come from a mind that is *untamed.* The eighth-century Buddhist saint Shantideva compares this untamed mind to a mad and drunken elephant that tramples everything in its path. The mind follows past habits, anticipates the future, and in the present gets entangled and lost in whatever thoughts and emotions happen to arise. Left to its own devices, it can lead us into intense suffering. However, if we can tame or conquer our minds, then nothing can frighten or upset us. The Buddha explained that anxiety, fear, and suffering only arise in minds that are in the grip of delusion and distraction. In other words, there is nothing to fear *except* our own untamed mind.[1]

With our body, our speech, and our mind, we generate actions, words, and thoughts, positive or negative, and sow the seeds of their future consequences, whatever they may be. Yet, on close examination, we can see that the most important of these three components of our being is the mind, and the body and the speech are merely its servants. To put it simply, the mind is the boss. This is why, in the Tibetan teachings, mind is called "the king who is responsible for everything"—*kun jé gyalpo*—the universal ordering principle.

As Buddha said:

> We are what we think.
> All that we are arises with our thoughts.

With our thoughts we make the world.
Speak or act with an impure mind
And trouble will follow you
As the wheel follows the ox that draws the cart.
We are what we think.
All that we are arises with our thoughts.
With our thoughts we make the world.
Speak or act with a pure mind
And happiness will follow you
As your shadow, unshakable.[2]

In the same spirit, Shakespeare made Hamlet say: "There is nothing either good or bad, but thinking makes it so."[3]

The mind, then, is the root of everything—the creator of happiness and the creator of suffering, the creator of what we call *samsara* and what we call *nirvana*. The Sanskrit word *samsara* means the cycle of existence, of birth and death, characterized by suffering and determined by our destructive emotions and our harmful actions. *Nirvana* means "the state beyond suffering and sorrow"; it can be said to be the state of buddhahood or enlightenment itself.

There is a verse by Shantideva that I find acutely moving, and devastatingly true:

Though longing to be happy, in their ignorance,
They destroy their own well-being, as if it were their worst
    enemy.
Although they long to be rid of suffering,
They rush headlong towards suffering itself.[4]

That is samsara in a nutshell. Even though we want happiness, we seem to do everything we can to heap suffering upon ourselves. Our aims and our actions are completely at odds. But, to be clear, life itself is not samsara; samsara is the confused and deluded way we choose to live. Lacking the wisdom of discernment, we let our destructive emotions, such as craving, anger, or ignorance, drive us toward harmful and unwholesome actions. The result is suffering, both for ourselves and for others.

If we know how to use this mind of ours, and if we come to understand our mind and its true nature, then nothing is more wonderful. We become the master of our own self, and our mind becomes the source of freedom. Unfortunately, if we don't know how to use the mind, and we are dominated by our thoughts and disturbing emotions, then the mind can prove our very worst enemy, a real nightmare. The poet Milton summed this up in *Paradise Lost*:

> The mind is its own place, and in itself
> Can make a Heaven of Hell, a Hell of Heaven.[5]

To know that the mind is the root of everything is to realize that we are ultimately responsible for both our own happiness and our own suffering. It is in our hands. And, as we are discovering more and more today, although the mind may contribute to ill health, it also possesses an extraordinary power of healing. What this means is that happiness and wholeness are completely attainable and completely within our reach.

The Appearance and the Essence of Mind

Now, if we say that the mind is the creator of samsara and nirvana, you might well ask: "What kind of mind creates samsara? What kind of mind creates nirvana?" This question may be the most important of our entire life. And the answer is revolutionary. It is the key to everything.

The great Tibetan master Tulku Urgyen Rinpoche would often explain:

> Samsara is mind turned outwardly, lost in its projections;
> Nirvana is mind turned inwardly, recognizing its true nature.

If someone were to ask us, "What is mind?" most of us would say, "My thoughts, my emotions, and my feelings." But according to the teachings of Buddha, these make up only one aspect of the mind. The teachings tell us that the mind has two aspects: the appearance of mind and, more important, the essence or nature of mind. His Holiness the Dalai Lama often describes these two aspects as "appearance and reality." All those thoughts and emotions are merely the appearances of mind, like the rays of light streaming from the sun. Then there is the very nature of mind, like the sun itself in all its glory. This is the all-important understanding.

As long as we are lost in mind's projections and appearances, we have no idea what this essence of mind might be. Mistakenly, we identify with thoughts and emotions, and take them to be all that we are. So if we have a positive thought, we conclude that we are good, and if we have a mean thought, we condemn ourselves as terrible and unworthy. We make such a big deal about our thoughts, we take them so seriously and we concoct all sorts of stories, which we believe are real and solid, and hold on to for dear life. But in the end, they are just the products of our mind. They dissolve, and they are gone. Ask yourself: Where are all the thoughts you had this morning? They don't exist. They were fleeting, impermanent, and constantly changing. And does anyone see these thoughts of yours? Do you? They just come and they go, but we attach such huge importance to them. They arise and settle all on their own, quite naturally, just like the waves that arise and then settle, back into the ocean. As the great Indian Buddhist master Tilopa told his disciple Naropa:

> It's not the appearances that bind you, but the grasping.
> Therefore abandon grasping, Naropa, my son.

We can think of these appearances, the thoughts and emotions, as being like clouds, whereas the true nature of our mind is like the sky. Even though the clouds may cover the sky, if you take a plane and fly up way beyond them, you will find an infinite expanse of clear blue sky that is never touched by the clouds. In the same way, the thoughts and emotions are not really our mind; they just go drifting by, like the clouds. It's all a question of our perspective: whether we view the thoughts and emotions the way the sky views the clouds, or we view them like someone down on the ground looking up and unable even to believe there is a sky up there beyond the clouds.

We need to remind ourselves that thoughts and emotions are only *one* aspect of mind but not the mind itself, nor the most important aspect. The more we dwell on our thoughts and emotions, trying to figure them out or search for answers, the more we find that peace of mind will elude us. So don't try to understand all your thoughts and emotions; there is simply no end to them. It's as if you send a friend to look for someone, your friend gets lost, and you have to send a second person to look for them, and then a third . . . and so on. Besides, by dwelling on the mind's projections and appearances, we are simply looking in the wrong direction, as if we were facing west and waiting for the sun to rise. As the great Tibetan master Patrul Rinpoche wrote, "It's like leaving your elephant at home and looking for its footprints in the forest." Instead of looking for the elephant itself, we go chasing after its footprints—our thoughts and emotions—and all that achieves is to take us further and further away from ourselves, and the true nature of our mind.

The ancient Greeks had a saying, "Know thyself," which was inscribed in the temple at Delphi. To know yourself is to know and understand the essence and nature of the mind. This is our most important task in life. Padmasambhava, the great master who established the Buddha's teachings in Tibet in the eighth or ninth century, said:

> Don't try to get to the root of everything:
> Go straight to the root of the mind.
> Once you get to the root of the mind,

You'll know the one thing that liberates all.
If you fail to fathom the root of the mind,
You can know everything, but understand nothing.

Our mind is a curious thing. At one moment it can be argumentative, opinionated, restless, and teeming with so many thoughts and emotions that we could just go crazy. But if you know how to just turn your mind inward, in the very next moment the thoughts and emotions all suddenly dissolve and evaporate. In a matter of seconds, the mind can be totally transformed. When we talk about "turning the mind inward," it does not mean becoming introverted or withdrawn; it simply means that we no longer let our mind get lost in thought and emotion and go on projecting outward. It means allowing the mind to be in its natural state: just turning slightly inward, to look into the face of its true nature.

What is amazing is that the moment you let go of projecting outward, and you turn your mind inward, something quite extraordinary can happen. And so my master Dilgo Khyentse Rinpoche used to say,

Do not let your mind be distracted.
Look, directly, at its very nature.

Because all along, the crucial point is *where* exactly your mind is, or the direction in which it is facing: whether it is outwardly looking, lost in thoughts and emotions, or inwardly seeing, recognizing its true nature.

Our mind is like a crystal; its fundamental essence or nature is always pure, pristine, and unchanging. But just as a crystal adopts the color of whatever surface you place it on, red or green, the mind will become just whatever we allow to occupy it, be it compassion, anger, or desire.

It is how we think or perceive that defines our reality. So if we can tame, transform, and conquer our mind, then we will transform our own perceptions and our whole experience, and, as a result, even circumstances and outer appearances will begin to change and appear differently.

I remember a discussion a few years ago between the Dalai Lama and Aaron T. Beck, the founder of cognitive therapy. It seemed to make a profound impression on His Holiness. Dr. Beck explained that, in his personal experience, when we have a strong outburst of emotion—anger, for example—90 percent of the time we mask reality by adding to it all our prejudices and our distorted view of things. His Holiness agreed, saying that even though there might be some basis for us to see a given situation as positive or negative, we exaggerate the "good" or "bad" aspect, and that causes us to respond with strong attachment or anger.[6]

Whenever we see a situation from the point of view of anger, then, we can say that there is 90 percent mental projection, and only 10 percent that really corresponds to reality. On the other hand, if our mind is calm and peaceful, it will be much easier for us to remain objective and to see reality as it is.

Usually, however, our minds are scattered everywhere and, as I like to say, "Nobody's at home." We are always *doing* things, always speaking and always thinking, but we have no idea of the doer, no idea of the speaker, and no idea of the thinker. More often than not, we don't even know, or maybe we never did, the purpose behind what we are doing. We simply do things by rote. And if we're not busy and our schedules are not full, we are almost embarrassed.

We have lost something immeasurably precious: our sense of being. We don't know how to just be, without any agenda. This is why we cannot find contentment. The French philosopher Pascal wrote, "All of man's difficulties are caused by his inability to sit, quietly, in a room by himself."[7] It's true: We are plagued by a sense of restlessness; speed and aggression dominate our lives. We don't know how to settle in ourselves, come in touch with ourselves, and find our ground.

We need to learn how to be.

Meditation and Its Methods

There are many ways to describe meditation. You can say that meditation is bringing the mind home, or getting to know our own mind, or coming to understand and work with the mind. You can say meditation is a process of overcoming the appearances of thoughts and emotions, and of coming slowly to enter the nature of mind. Through the practice of meditation we can break free from our fixation on thoughts and emotions, and begin to develop the capacity to remain more in the essence and nature of mind, rather than in its endless variety of appearances. The practice of meditation also gives our mind stability. At the same time, meditation awakens in us a deep feeling of well-being, which is one of the reasons why it is so beneficial for our physical and mental health.

Meditation can be presented as a subject both vast—with its various stages and levels—and extremely profound. But the basics of meditation are actually very simple, and so there is no cause to feel daunted or overwhelmed. Anyone can meditate, anyone at all, and you can do it almost anywhere and at any time.

The first and most fundamental practice of meditation is to allow the mind to settle into a state of "calm abiding," where it will find peace and stability and can rest in a state of nondistraction. This type of meditation is known as *shamatha* in Sanskrit, and *shyiné* in Tibetan. When you first begin to meditate, you may use a support: for example, looking at an object or an image of Buddha, or Christ if you are a Christian practitioner; using a mantra or chant; or lightly, mindfully watching the breath, which is common to all spiritual traditions.[8] In time, you can also use anything you experience through your five senses as a support or object for meditation, anything you see, hear, taste, smell, or touch, as well as any thoughts or emotions you may be experiencing. This approach is known as "shamatha with support."

The purpose of any of these methods is to help the mind remain undistracted. All of them lead to the same result. If you are using the breath as the support for your practice, you focus your mind ever so lightly, and mindfully, on the breath. When you are breathing out, just know that you are breathing out; when you breathe in, know that you are breathing in. No other thought, concept, or commentary is required, because apart from pure knowing, nothing else is involved. There is no analysis and no conceptualization but simply pure knowing, pure mindfulness, and pure awareness.

So the discipline is to keep bringing your mind back to the breath. If you are distracted, then the instant you remember, you simply bring your mind back to the breath. Nothing else is necessary. Even asking yourself, "How on earth did I get so distracted?" is only another distraction. The simplicity of mindfulness, of continuously returning your mind to the breath or whatever you are using as the object of your meditation practice, gradually calms it down.

There is an example that I am fond of. When you are trying to put an infant to bed, she will want to start to play, and if you give in, she will get more and more excited, and never go to sleep. The trick is that you have to hold her and stay with her quietly, and eventually she will calm down. Mind is just the same: at first it may be very jumpy. But however agitated it gets, keep bringing it back, time and time again, to the simplicity of breathing. Gradually, mind will settle, in the mind. And you will know more how to be.

As I wrote in *The Tibetan Book of Living and Dying*:

> What is very important, the masters always advise, is not to fixate while practicing the concentration of calm abiding. That is why they recommend you place only 25 percent of your attention on mindfulness of the breath. But then, as you may have noticed, mindfulness alone is not enough. While you are supposed to be watching the breath, after a few minutes you may find yourself playing in a football match or starring in your own movie. So another 25 percent should be devoted to a continuous and watchful awareness, one that oversees and checks whether you are being mindful of the breath. The remaining 50 percent of your attention is left abiding, spaciously.[9]

Of course, the exact percentages are not as important as the fact that all three of these elements—mindfulness, awareness, and spaciousness—are present.

Gradually, with practice, you will find that you are able to rest your mind, undistracted and aware, in the present moment, without needing to focus on any particular support or object. At that point you can drop the method altogether and practice what is called "shamatha without support." You might wonder how you can rest your mind without a support. All you need to do is simply let go, relax, and leave your mind, undistracted, maintaining the barest attention to the present moment. You rest in a state of pure knowing, aware of everything that passes through your mind. Whatever thoughts, emotions, and feelings come, neither do you try to block them nor do you follow them. They come and go, like the wind. The secret is not to think about them but allow them to flow through the mind, while keeping your mind free of "afterthoughts."

As you rest in this awareness, it dawns on you that you are much bigger than your thoughts, emotions, and perceptions. At the same time you realize that you don't have to be afraid of your thoughts. Because thoughts are *not you*. Emotions are *not you*. You can become free of them, and the more you do so, the more you come in touch with the confidence of your true nature, and start to become the master of your own mind.

Finally, let's take a brief glance at meditation at the deepest level. At its most profound, meditation is simply resting in the very nature of the mind, without manipulating, contriving, or altering anything at all. There is a wonderful saying by the great masters of the past. I remember when I first heard it what a revelation it was, because in these two lines is shown not only what the nature of mind is but also how to bring it into our experience and abide by it, which is the practice of meditation at the highest level. In Tibetan it is very beautiful, with an almost musical lilt:

chu ma nyok na dang
sem ma chö na dé

It means, roughly translated,

Water, if you don't stir it, will become clear;
The mind, left unaltered, will find its own natural peace,
well-being, happiness, and bliss.

What I find so striking about this instruction is its emphasis on naturalness, on allowing our mind simply to be, unaltered, without changing anything at all. There is not the slightest trace of contrivance, fabrication, or manipulation. Because the trouble with our mind is that we are always fabricating, always contriving, always manipulating through thinking.

The great Tibetan master Longchenpa said:

Do not alter, do not alter,
Do not alter this mind of ours.
Do not grasp, do not grasp,
Do not grasp at this mind of ours.
Alter and alter, and you will stir up the cloudy depths of the mind,
And a mind that is altered obscures its own true nature.[10]

What is truly extraordinary is that *not altering* our mind brings about in us the greatest change of all. We carry around such a long history of getting caught up in our thoughts and emotions that we assume it must be almost impossible to arrive at the nature of mind, but actually it is available to us immediately. In a matter of seconds we can discover the peace of our true nature. It is then that we begin to realize that this peace is with us all the time, and is never apart from us.

Then, too, we will have discovered the true and ultimate purpose of meditation, which is to awaken in us the sky-like nature of mind, and to introduce us to the unchanging pure awareness that underlies the whole of our experience. Once I described it like this:

As our cloud-like thoughts and emotions fade away, the sky-like expanse of our true being is revealed, and, shining from it, our true nature, which is like the sun. And just as both light and warmth blaze from the sun, wisdom and loving compassion radiate out from the mind's innermost nature. Grasping at a false self, or ego, has dissolved, and we simply rest, as much as we can, in the nature of mind, this most natural state which is without any reference or concept, hope or fear, yet with a quiet but soaring confidence—the deepest form of well-being imaginable.[11]

Meditation and Well-Being

Earlier I touched upon the importance of inner peace and deep, mental contentment and their power to transform our lives. Real contentment comes, as we have seen, by not getting lost in the stories and projections, by turning the mind inward, and by rediscovering that lost sense of "simply being." Then you become, it is said, like an old, wise man watching a child play. Without any need to follow or believe in your thoughts and emotions, you simply remain relaxed and aware of everything that flits through your mind, just as it is. You are completely unperturbed and unaffected by whatever comes up. And as you watch yourself, and spot how readily your mind turns outward, and spins one story line after another, you might even smile and laugh gently at yourself, amused by how ridiculous and absurd your mind can be, especially in the light of whatever you have understood of the essence and nature of the mind.

Research into the impact of meditation is constantly revealing its wonderful healing effects on our mind and body. As the mind settles in the practice of meditation, something extraordinary seems to take place. For a start, our restless, thinking mind subsides into a state of deep inner peace, the scattered, fragmented aspects of ourselves come home, and we can become whole. Those contradictory voices, dictates, and feelings that fight for control over our inner lives settle and become friends, the pain and distress of struggling with ourselves dissolve, and a deep and compassionate forgiveness of ourselves becomes possible. Overall, we notice that with regular meditation practice, negativity is undone, speed and aggression are pacified, frustration, tension, and turbulent emotions are defused, and the unkindness, violence, and harm in us are removed, revealing our inherent "good heart," the fundamental goodness and kindness that is our true nature. This is why I always say meditation is real "inner disarmament."

Also, as more and more researchers are telling us these days, with regular meditation practice we tend to enjoy greater physical well-being and better health. We become "well in our own skin," we are content and happy with who we are, and we feel more self-confidence, self-esteem, and self-worth. Then, quite naturally, the more we get in touch with who *we* really are through meditation, the more we can be completely in touch with *others,* too. Difficult people and situations that otherwise might have caused us harm or posed a huge problem are softened and easier to deal with. Conflicts are resolved, and we find we are more likely to be in harmony with others, and naturally easier to get along with—because our minds are relatively free and uncomplicated—and we turn out to be quite good company!

With meditation practice, the environment of our mind and heart transforms, and with that, our outer environment can change as well, so that wherever we are, we can find contentment and happiness and begin to see the beauty in ordinary things. And as we gradually integrate meditation into our everyday life, and mindfulness and awareness begin to permeate our actions, words, and thoughts, there builds in us a certain simplicity, stability, confidence, and readiness with which we can meet life and the complexity of the world with composure, compassion, ease, and humor.

2

Meditation Methods in the Buddhist Tradition

Jetsün Khandro Rinpoche

Meditation may be less of a mystery today than it once was, but do we really understand its true purpose? And what on earth does it have to do with cotton balls, donkeys, and carrots? The eminent Tibetan Buddhist teacher Jetsün Khandro Rinpoche begins by explaining the origins of the word meditation, *and how it leads us to the personal responsibility we have for shaping our inner and outer world. In the silence and stillness of meditation, we come to challenge our usual ways of seeing things and uncover the tremendous capacity and potential that we all possess.*

I am going to discuss the two things that matter most to human beings: medicine and—I would love to say Buddhism, but let's keep it general—spiritual philosophy.

Meditation is a very commonly heard word today, so much so that when we say it, people have all kinds of ideas of what it might be. They range from stereotypical images of ascetics meditating in the Himalayan mountains, sages standing or lying on beds of nails, or people remaining in a mummified position in deep caves without eating or speaking for many years, to soccer or baseball teams doing meditation before a game, prisoners following meditation programs in prisons, or beauty salons where you can do a therapeutic meditation before getting a facial. Oprah Winfrey is talking about meditation. His Holiness the Dalai Lama is speaking about meditation. We have a wide range of usages of the word. This has brought us to a point where people come to meditation or do not come to meditation because of these preconceived assumptions of what meditation is.

Although there are positive results of widespread knowledge of any concept, there is also a downside, if we do not explore the subject more directly and instead accept our preconceived assumptions of what it might be.

Given the variety of concepts about what meditation is, let us begin by looking at the literal meaning of the word. From a Buddhist perspective, meditation originally derives from the Sanskrit term *samadhi*. If we dissect the literal meaning of this term, we come to a much simpler meaning: maintaining a state of detached equilibrium—a state of equilibrium, balance, or equanimity but with the quality of detachment.

Detachment doesn't mean "throw it away" or "don't have feelings about it." It definitely does not mean denying, or obstructing the mind's natural tendency to project. Imagine you are about to go into a cotton factory. Before entering you pour glue all over your body, and then you demand, "I don't want any cotton balls to stick to my body, but I won't remove the glue from my body either." Then you enter the cotton factory. Of course the glue, by its nature, makes cotton balls stick to you. In meditative language, that kind of stickiness is called deliberation or fabrication, and here we call it the state of nondetachment. The state of nondetachment is when you get entangled and you make the story line similar to that of a daytime soap opera in which four characters go on for twenty years. It keeps on multiplying and you exaggerate the situation.

You create a state in your mind that is full of grasping, clinging, and attachment.

From a meditative point of view, samadhi means to bring about a situation in your mind that allows a state of resting within detached equilibrium. The Tibetan word we use for the same concept is *ting nge dzin*. It can be literally translated as "remaining in a state of concentration," or "holding concentration." Holding concentration without fixation. Colloquially we use the word *gom*, which today is very easily translated as meditation, but *gom* literally means "familiarity," not "meditation." If we take time to contemplate these expressions—"creating a state within oneself that is a continuum of balance of awareness," "becoming familiar with remaining in a state of detached equilibrium," or "becoming familiar with maintaining a focus or concentration without fixation"—it will be much easier to understand what we mean by meditation.

Meditation has nothing to do with spirituality per se. Many scholars will beg to differ with me when I say this. If you investigate meditation carefully, however, it really doesn't. Let me share a story that has stayed with me my whole life. As children growing up in a Tibetan refugee community in Northern India, we used to get many nice storybooks donated so that we could read and learn English. Of all these books, my favorites were a series about Clever Monkey and his friend Stupid Donkey. In one of the stories Stupid Donkey decides to enter a horse race. Everyone tries to convince Stupid Donkey that he will not win the race, saying, "You're a donkey, and on top of that you're really stupid. You're just going to embarrass yourself!" Clever Monkey, in particular, tries to discourage his friend Stupid Donkey, but the Stupid Donkey absolutely insists on running the race, and gets in line ready for the start. The race begins, but Stupid Donkey does not move because his nature is to be stubborn. All the donkey's friends try to get him to move. Finally Clever Monkey comes up with an idea. He hops onto Stupid Donkey's back and holds out a fishing rod with a bunch of carrots dangling in front of the donkey's face. The donkey sees the bunch of carrots and gains the inspiration to try to get them, but as he moves forward, the fishing rod moves forward, and the carrots move forward. Stupid Donkey ultimately wins the race, not because of the race itself but because of the bunch of carrots.

With deep respect to all spiritual leaders, I have learned over time that religion and spirituality are like the bunch of carrots. The whole point of the race is to make human beings civilized and enable them to generate awareness of their own inner potential. But our wise species known as human beings, the most intelligent of all living species—would we do things simply? Are we not like the very stubborn donkey? Until we find a result, something to get, a profit to make, something that would make us compete and gain victory, would we actually do things simply? No.

So the great, kind masters, like the wise monkey, come up with the wonderful idea of a bunch of carrots on a fishing rod. Some call it heaven, some call it enlightenment, some call it virtue, some call it merit, some call it *bodhisattvas*, angels, divine powers, energies—it does not matter. Just race, finally win the race, and get the carrot, whatever that carrot might represent.

If we look at it from this perspective, it is possible to approach meditation as something a lot less threatening. You do not find yourself in a position where you are seduced to meditate. Instead, you understand that from the Buddhist philosophical perspective, it does not matter whether you call it meditation or a continuum of balance that you create in your mind. The most important thing is that you are able to recognize this tremendous inner power and capacity that you are endowed with, and that you spend time with it. If you feel inspired calling it meditation, then that is what is meditation. Many of us would not meditate, and would not wake up to our inner potential, were it not given to us in the form of the teachings of the enlightened Buddha, were it not a philosophy which our dearly loved teachers teach. On the other hand, many people could do it without all this paraphernalia. That is absolutely fine, too, and of all the people who would not mind a bit, the first one would be the Buddha himself.

Having said that, if we go by the literal meaning of the term *meditation*, it requires us to be aware of our inner potential. There are countless different techniques and methods of Buddhist meditation. In fact, there are as many different particular types of meditation as there are individuals. That is what makes this whole system very dependent on what is known as the teacher–student relationship. It is not about a holy relationship. It is about exact knowledge. A doctor and patient have the confidentiality, trust, and complete connectedness and understanding that allow them to meet for five minutes and speak volumes. Meditation technique requires the same kind of relationship: the teacher knows the student and the student knows the teacher well enough so that the student can work with his own self and depend less on external factors. The student gets to the point of realizing that he is working on the development of the inner power of his mind.

Meditation is widely spoken of these days, and there are many well-known meditation methods. These include the very simple breathing techniques of *pranayama,* which originate in the ancient Indian civilization and the traditions of yoga. There is *shamatha,* usually called placement meditation, resting meditation, or meditation of simply abiding and resting. Another well-known method is *vipassana.* One type of vipassana is described in terms of a resultant state, which is more of a settling vipassana. Then there are much more causal vipassana meditations, which have more of a flavor of investigation and examination.

In Mahayana Buddhism, and particularly in the Tibetan Buddhist tradition, we have an even greater variety of methods, all of them unique and powerful. Some of them are evocative meditations that deal with visualization and creation. There are deconstructive meditations, called dissolution meditations, where you deconstruct every projection to finally investigate its true nature. There are what we call peaceful methods of meditation, as well as wrathful forms of meditation. There are sound meditations, thought meditations, and non-thought meditations. These are the methods of Buddhist meditation that would be listed in any number of books that you can get.

The essence of what all these methods are trying to teach us is basically what foggy, rainy weather teaches us. Instead of emphasizing the external projection, move inward. We all know that outside there is a beautiful environment, with trees, mountains, roads, meadows, and fields; and yet we know we are inside. Taking that as an example of what meditation is trying to teach, all of these techniques are oriented toward dismantling a very stubborn, habitual belief in concepts that we human beings have created. As I mentioned earlier, science describes human beings as the most brilliant of all species, but brilliance can sometimes become its own worst enemy. We have the capacity of being able to see things, but our seeing things may lead to an extremely stubborn attitude, to a blame game where external concepts are blamed as the causes of our experiences.

We also have the capacity to hear and articulate sounds, yet the habit of hearing sounds may create in us a stubborn attitude of always blaming sounds as external. This leads us to come up with such illogical notions as "good sounds" versus "bad sounds." If there were no notion of good sound or bad sound, we would not have feelings of aversion or attachment toward the things we hear.

It is the same with our senses of taste and smell, our body, which feels textures, and, most important, our mind, which comes up with all kinds of different thoughts. It is a wonderful potential that we are all naturally gifted with, yet that gift becomes intertwined with two things. I would like to say "ego," but let's use some less Buddhist terminology and call it "stubbornness." This attitude of stubbornness is joined with another aspect of the human temperament, which is being very quick and impatient. Since we are always impatient and we are going to be stubborn, we have to find quick answers to everything, and the quickest answer seems to be to segregate everything into things we like and things we do not like. So we have developed a habit of always saying, "This is what I like, and this is what I do not like." What you do not like is blamed for a number of experiences that you go through in life. What you do like you can never get enough of. Half of your life is spent chasing after that, and the other half is spent running away from what you do not want to encounter. These are what we consider sensible activities in the life of the most brilliant of species.

The Buddha called it suffering. The Buddhist philosophy of creation of suffering and the causes and conditions that lead to suffering is not taught for the sake of being profound but because it is just what we do. Suffering is not just about blood and tears, death and dying, and impermanence. These are simpler sufferings. The most complex feature of suffering is that we are capable of addressing it but we do not do it, we complain that we do not do it, and we complain some more. This just cannot be justified, especially when we simultaneously claim to be the most brilliant of all species. If that is not suffering, what is? It is a very sad story, because from just that one point we create this world, we lead this world, and we are responsible for the generations to come and how they will live life in this world.

Meditation and the techniques of meditation point to the individual responsibility of every human being. From that perspective, the more one meditates, the more one will recognize one's own inner potential, inner qualities, and inner capabilities. But while meditation is trying to look into the senses, the short-temperedness and quick judgments that our mind makes, and the impatient and stubborn attitude with which it relates to the senses, from the Buddhist perspective it is important to examine the causes of these judgments and attitudes.

You create causes of happiness or suffering because of what your senses perceive, and how you articulate these perceptions, particularly in the form of thoughts that propel you to create actions of the body and in speech. Causes and conditions are created because you are active with your body, speech, and mind. Through meditation, you realize the inner responsibility of seeing that to obtain the resultant state of goodness, health, or well-being—or you could call it enlightenment—you must be very aware of causes.

Simply intending to create correct causes, however, will not make it happen. Therefore, meditators are taught that the method of meditation is to dismantle habitual ways of making concrete concepts. We are taught how important it is for us to spend time in inner contemplation, to see whether or not things are as we have assumed them to be in the quickness of our habits of judgments and opinions. Making concepts very solid and concrete, and on that basis forming quick judgments and quick opinions, is very familiar to us. It is convenient and is so familiar that it does not take much effort.

I have often felt that it is similar to having an old pair of shoes that are really wearing out. You know that if you keep wearing them, they will give you bad knees and a bad back, so you go out and buy an expensive new pair of shoes. But when it comes to walking, which shoes do you choose, the old pair or the new pair? You choose the old pair of shoes, because you know how they will fit. You know there is a bump there, a dent here, and a tear here and there, but at the same time the familiarity of knowing what you will experience, even if it will ultimately turn out to be painful, is far more comforting to you than risking wearing that expensive pair of shoes that took two hours to find, that you should be wearing, and that will be good for you and your back. Habits are like that. Solidifying concepts is a habit—we are used to doing this. Coming up with a quick thought—*this is good, that is bad*—is so much easier. That is why meditation has never been very popular: it asks you to reverse a process that you have been living by your whole life. So until a person recognizes that it is really important to break this habit, I believe that she will be skeptical of meditation.

As I have outlined, Buddhist meditation techniques are varied and it can be a complex topic, requiring lifetimes to explore. At the same time, if we view meditation as a method for breaking down habitual ways of looking at things and for looking at things in a slightly different way, then all different techniques of meditation can be broken down into three simple points: working with body, speech, and mind.

Prior to going into formal meditation, I feel a very good preliminary process, particularly if you do not have any previous experience of meditation, is to begin with a simple notion of "observance" or "watchfulness." Traditionally all meditation techniques have been introduced with the same line: "Find a place of solitude"—a quiet place where people are not coming and going—and sit comfortably. You are told to find a place of solitude so that you can really work against being self-conscious about your meditation. If you meditate wanting others to see how wonderfully you are meditating, it is a wrong, forced approach. You will never get to naturalness by being self-conscious.

Even if you do not belong to the category of people who like others to feel inspired by your meditation, there are people who like to meditate for *themselves*. If you are such a person and you are surrounded by people when you meditate, you will feel self-conscious inwardly. You will be very conscious of people looking at you. Let's say you are trying to be in your natural state and there are two people watching you and commenting on you, pointing fingers and shaking their heads. It makes it very difficult to get down to meditation. Therefore, in the beginning, allow yourself to enjoy being alone. Being alone is a good way to start being totally without pretense. With pretentiousness and any kind of deliberation or self-consciousness, you have deviated from finding what your natural, true nature is, into what you would like the natural, true nature to look like. That is the moment when you bring spirituality into meditation. Even as a Buddhist, if you bring a Buddhist flavor to it you have basically made your journey very long for yourself.

For this reason it is important to keep it very simple and learn to be observant and watchful. Find a place for yourself where you can be watchful and observant, avoiding both the extremes. One, as you watch yourself, do not always find reasons and excuses. Let's say you watch yourself and you have a thought. Do not follow having watched and observed the thought by commending yourself. It is not necessary for you to support the thought, or to find reasons and excuses why that thought should be generated. At the same time, avoid the other extreme—much more an obstacle in the case of seasoned meditators—which is cynicism and critical ideas about thoughts. After years and years of learning to meditate, I remember going to my teacher and saying, "These thoughts just won't cease!" My teacher turned to me and said, "They will when you die! A corpse has no thoughts. Get on with it."

It is important to keep that very direct approach in mind and to know that thoughts are a natural expression of a very vivid, clear mind. While thoughts are arising, it is clearly okay for you as an observer, as somebody watching, not to go to the extreme of generating opinions and judgments. Instead, become educated and thoroughly introduced to how vivid your mind is. You will never be able to train that elusive mind through meditation if you do not first recognize what it is that you are working with. Because it is completely invisible, and yet so full of power and energy, capacities, and capabilities, it is a very complex thing. And the best way to know it, the best way to introduce yourself to it, is by watching it and by being observant.

The first result of looking at your own vividness (whether you call it mind, consciousness, thoughts, mental patterns, emotions, feelings, concepts—it really does not matter, because they are all the same) and at the influx of immense creativity you are generating should be that you become introduced to the great, vivid, and vibrant nature of mind, and that you understand the power of the mind. You begin to realize that a lot of the things you are dealing with in life are all based upon perception. You are perceiving things, and how you perceive things and how you articulate what you perceive is often going to be the causal basis of how you will bring out the colors of your life.

As a child I was educated at a Catholic convent in Northern India. At the first class I attended, our priest pointed to a glass of water on a table and said, "What do you see? Do you see a glass half full or a glass half empty?" We were all told to say, "I see the glass half full"—to have a very positive outlook on life. It was a wonderful and classic example of perspective, of how you are trained to perceive things. Mind is your intrinsic power and its expressivity lies in perceptions. Your happiness is a perception, it is how you perceive things. Not knowing that, we often blame concepts, thoughts, and external things for our emotions. But if you observe how much you could articulate every concept, feeling, and emotion as it arises from within, you almost become an artist with varied colored paintbrushes in your hands and a blank canvas in front of you. You can splash it with rainbows of color, you can paint it dark and bleak, you can make it all black, all white, or a multitude of colors. That is the power of mind and perception.

If our perception is so important, how can we influence the way we perceive things? We cloud our perception by not allowing it the space and the freedom to become more vivid, clear, and awake. That is where a method of meditation might be helpful. There is a wonderful metaphor of providing a large, open field for cows to graze in. This is precisely what we are talking about. Allowing your perception to have more spaciousness and openness is where you are able to bring in the three crucial points of stillness, silence, and non-thought. Within these three points of stillness, silence, and non-thought is a summation of all the different kinds of meditation methods: analytical, placement, peaceful, wrathful, investigative, evocative, experiential, and many others.

Stillness is the foundation, wherever you are and whatever you might be doing—from traditional sitting still in meditation to a stillness of the body as you go for a walk. Stillness is not only a physical posture of sitting down in a certain place, but it is being observant of your body, so that the body is able to contain this very powerful mind in a much more nurtured and protected environment of awareness.

The first meditation technique from which everyone could

benefit is to allow yourself to be still for a long time. If possible, start with at least fifteen minutes. Anything shorter than that would be just an experiment that might give you a quick fix, but as they say, there is no shortcut to realizing your own fundamental nature. And you have to have the humility to recognize that you are actually reversing the current. In my case, let's say it is forty-two years of action-engaged body versus fifteen minutes of stillness. Which one is going to win? Which one will I be more familiar with? You need to know what your habit is, and what you are reversing. Each day try to find stillness. Sit still. There is nothing Buddhist, meditative, or spiritual about it. You are just allowing your body, which contains a powerful mind, to be given some rejuvenation time, some respite. You are giving yourself some spaciousness to sit and, in that stillness, to discover the incredibly vivid and vibrant quality of the mind.

This discovery comes in the form of the stillness being intertwined with silence—silence of the verbal speech as well as silence of the mental chatter that is happening all the time. Having disciplined yourself to sit quietly, first cut down on verbal speech and then cut down on mental chatter. Tell yourself, "I do deserve fifteen minutes of peace and quiet. I do deserve a moment when I can relax into not having to think of something fantastic, into not having to articulate and have opinions and judgments." If you are still not sure, I like to remind meditators that after these fifteen minutes, things will still be the same. You can continue; nothing will have changed. So without the fear that something drastic is going to happen, give yourself the time to sit quietly in physical stillness and verbal silence.

Through the habit and familiarity with this mental, verbal, and physical quietude, you will realize the state called non-thought. As I said earlier, non-thought means not following, not grasping, and remaining quite detached, like a person who walks into a cotton factory without being covered in glue. Allow the splendor of all the cotton balls and all the activity happening around you, but just be by yourself, within yourself, at that moment. Through the stillness and silence, create a state of watching the enormous display of every activity your senses provide, while at the same time remaining detached from formulating opinions and judgments about it.

When silence, stillness, and non-thought become a foundation you build within yourself, it opens the gateway to the very acute, direct understanding of what we call looking at the inner mind, or working with one's deeper inherent nature. Until then the deeper inherent nature continues to be like clouds and mists, and we do not seem to have the time to clear them and find out more, because we are so used to shortcuts, quick fixes, and quick results. We have a tremendous volume of opinions, ideas, and judgments, and then we insist that everybody should agree with them, and wonder why nobody is actually able to understand *my* problems. Suffering ensues from that.

Even though numerous philosophies and different world religions have tried to speak about this deeper inherent nature in different ways, it cannot be understood until we have a direct conviction of it. No multitude of philosophies is going to convince us to the degree where we would be willing to break free of our habitual ways of thinking until we gain a direct conviction ourselves. That conviction rests on experience, and experience cannot arise until you try it out for yourself.

This trying out is called the art of contemplation. Start with silence and stillness, and giving yourself a break for fifteen minutes each day. Whatever happens after you do this will become your own individual journey. If you stubbornly insist that your concepts are right and should be accepted, then welcome to the most complex philosophy in the world, Buddhist meditation. But if you really recognize that everything is dependent on the perception you have and how it unfolds, if you recognize your unique responsibility for how you engage in the perceptions you produce, then it becomes very simple and that is how the Buddha taught. For this reason we say that liberation is in your own hands, dependent entirely on how you look at it. You can look at it in a positive way or you can look at it in a very complicated way. It is entirely an individual choice, which has to be respected, and that is what has led to the complexities of today's philosophical teachings.

PART TWO

The Science of Meditation

3

The Benefits of Meditation

A Scientific Reality

Dr. Frédéric Rosenfeld

Just a few decades ago, the idea that health-care professionals might one day teach their patients how to meditate was pure fantasy. Frédéric Rosenfeld, a psychiatrist from Lyon, France, is one of many physicians around the world who now do just that. He outlines some of the most important discoveries and developments that have helped to establish this increasingly fruitful alliance of meditation with medicine and science, including key research findings, the success of mindfulness programs, and the work of the Mind and Life Institute.

I discovered meditation in 2001, at a ten-day *vipassana* retreat in eastern France. I was a psychiatry intern at the time, and the retreat marked a real turning point for me. It opened up avenues of thought beyond those that I already knew through psychoanalysis, cognitive behavioral therapy, and neuroscience. I discovered that Buddhism held real treasures, jewels that could help me, and my fellow humans, to feel better. I continued to practice and tried to find ways to bring meditation and health care together. These two worlds were clearly rich with an understanding that could be shared and even synthesized.

Nowadays, *to meditate* means to reflect, or to consider at length, but the etymology of the word shows that it has something in common with medicine. The two words come from the same root, the Latin verb *medeor,* meaning "I cure," or "I heal."

Multiple Perspectives

Broadly speaking, the many different schools of meditation share two components. The first is *shamatha* (sometimes, *samatha),* which can be translated as tranquillity, peace, or inner calm, either mental or physical. The second component of most meditation practices is *vipassana* (or *vipashyana*). In the ancient language of Pali, *vipassana* means penetrating insight, but we can also give it a more modern translation: mindfulness, observing things as they are, not as we would—or would not—like them to be. Beyond these two basic components, however, it is worth noting that there is no single way of meditating. *Meditation* should really be written in the plural, because there are so many meditations—different approaches, perspectives, and practices.

Take Taoism, for example. Taoism is a philosophical movement that began in China centuries ago. Taoism has influenced Chinese medicine and inspired different meditative techniques: tai chi, which has several styles; *qigong,* which itself is a system of medical exercises; and Taoist meditations based on physical postures and on regulating the chi, or inner air. Zen, which calls the Buddha the "Great Doctor," is a practice (or practices) of meditation, but also a medical practice, as we will see later. Another example is Hinduism, with all its different schools of yoga that originated in India and neighboring countries. Practices closer to Western culture, such as Christian prayers, can also be a form of meditation, and there are meditations in the Jewish tradition that work with the breath, just like those that originated in India and China.

Is Meditation a Form of Treatment?

The question that concerns us here is, Can meditation help us to feel better, physically or psychologically? A somewhat disappointing first answer is, We don't meditate in order to feel better. Why not? Because a serious meditator has no expectations. A person who practices vipassana while imagining *I'm going to get rid of my migraine* or *I'm sure this is going to be good for my back pain* would most likely provoke amusement or irritation on the part of the meditation teacher. Practicing meditation means expecting nothing other than what the present moment brings, so in this sense, meditation is not a type of treatment. It requires that you require nothing.

If we consider the question of how meditation can help us feel better from a different angle, the Buddha spoke about suffering in the first teaching he gave, at Benares in India. Suffering is something that we all experience when we are ill, so it's clear that Buddhism does concern the domain of medicine. I have already mentioned Taoism and its influence on Chinese medicine, and there, too, we are in the domain of medicine. Finally, yoga and Ayurvedic medicine aim to treat or unify body and mind, so our second answer contradicts the first by affirming that, yes, meditation is indeed a form of treatment!

There is a third possible answer to the question, and it comes from modern science, which has confirmed over the course of several decades that meditation does contribute to our physical and mental health. For more than eighty years now, scientists have been interested in meditation, first hesitantly and then with more and more enthusiasm. In the 1920s, a center offering yoga courses in Lonavla, a small town in the Indian state of Maharashtra, allowed Western physiologists to verify the effects of yoga on health. They observed that practicing hatha yoga could relieve high blood pressure and help people with an irregular heartbeat. It was good for respiration as well, especially for respiratory conditions such as asthma. It was at Lonavla, then, that the first seeds of the relationship between Western science and meditation were sown.

In the 1960s, advances in technology allowed Japanese scientists to attach electrodes to the heads of Zen meditators. The monk Taisen Deshimaru, who introduced Zen Buddhism to Europe, took part in these experiments. The scientists observed an interesting phenomenon. Ordinarily, anyone sitting next to an alarm clock gets used to the ticking sound after a few minutes, and falls asleep. The brain of a Zen practitioner, however, listens in a different way. Each tick is perceived as if it were the first. Zen meditation develops the freshness of the present moment, and each second arises and subsides in consciousness as if it were being lived for the very first time. This observation, which has been described in Zen writings for centuries, has been confirmed by neuroscience in the past few decades.

In the 1970s, Herbert Benson, a cardiologist who was one of the pioneers of mind/body medicine, trekked into the foothills of the Himalayas to study the connections between Western relaxation techniques and meditation. His discoveries established several common elements that he called the "big four," which almost all forms of relaxation share: (1) a calm environment; (2) muscular relaxation; (3) letting go, or a "let it happen" attitude; and (4) a focus on an object (a flame, the breath, a thought, a physical sensation, and so on).

Many subsequent scientific studies in different fields of medicine, physiology, and psychology have also shed light on the positive effects of meditation on health:

- Certain practices can lower high blood cholesterol levels.
- Qigong strengthens the immune system.
- Meditation has an anti-aging effect, as shown by the work of Sara Lazar.[1]
- Meditation, and mindfulness in particular, can benefit people who are suffering from rheumatism.

- Meditation relieves the symptoms of certain digestive disorders, such as irritable bowel syndrome.
- Mindfulness can accelerate the healing of certain skin disorders, such as psoriasis.
- Patients with Parkinson's disease tend to walk with short steps. Certain forms of tai chi practiced by patients in the early stages of the disease helped them to lengthen their steps.

Mindfulness and Its Applications

In 1979, Jon Kabat-Zinn developed a program that he called Mindfulness-Based Stress Reduction (MBSR), a masterful combination of three meditative techniques: Zen, vipassana, and hatha yoga. Kabat-Zinn defines mindfulness as the awareness that arises by paying attention on purpose, in the present moment, and nonjudgmentally. It requires effort and training to remain in the present moment, trying to avoid distractions relating to the past or the future, and refraining from judgment—which is perhaps the most difficult part of all. The traditional Buddhist word used for this state of mindfulness is "equanimity," which means not being devoured by the demons of attachment and aversion.

Mindfulness was initially intended for people suffering from stress, but its therapeutic uses have expanded over the years. Astonishingly, the benefits of MBSR have been shown to be almost identical to the benefits of all other kinds of meditation. I believe that all good psychiatrists, psychologists, and psychotherapists should practice mindfulness, in order to help us understand our patients better. Because it cultivates an "emptiness" of the mind, mindfulness practice can encourage therapists to refrain from pigeonholing patients according to the rigid categories that they may have learned in their training.

Looking beyond the health benefits, what does it mean to be mindful? I would say that it means to know oneself. For anyone who wants to be in good health, knowing oneself means, first of all, knowing what is happening in one's mind. If we imagine a person who is angry, his suffering is expressed through the thoughts boiling away in his head. *My boss still hasn't given me a raise* or *My neighbor doesn't respect me.* The longer a toxic thought remains undetected by the conscious mind, the more likely we are to fall victim to it. To be mindful, on the other hand, means to observe the flow of thoughts going on in our head, pleasant or painful, without becoming caught up in them.

Knowing oneself also means knowing one's emotions. One hundred and fifty years ago Charles Darwin described six emotions: surprise, sadness, disgust, fear, joy, and anger. Thanks to mindfulness, we can all know our emotions simply by observing them. In the case of the angry man, not only do his thoughts poison his mind, but his body is shaken physically by the emotion, which can be felt in a specific area. Being mindful means taking note of the emotions that inhabit our body without acting on them.

Finally, knowing oneself through mindfulness involves experimentation. As the Buddha himself said, "Ehipassika!"—"Come and see!" As part of a mindfulness program, we do exercises daily at home to *feel* the technique physically. During these exercises, we bring our attention to our thoughts and emotions, just as we would to any object of research. By practicing mindfulness, patients might notice that their experience is constructed on the basis of their thoughts and emotions. Finally, going beyond mindfulness itself, they will realize that their concept of "I" is nothing more than an aggregate that they have created. At that point, they are not too far away from enlightenment.

Some years after the appearance of MBSR, a number of psychology researchers became interested in the beneficial effects of meditation on depression, a global epidemic affecting young and old. What is particularly pernicious about depression is that the more depressive episodes you have, the more likely you are to suffer a future relapse. After a third depressive episode, the risk of relapse is considerable. Three psychologists, Zindel Segal, Mark Williams, and John Teasdale, skillfully brought mindfulness together with cognitive behavioral therapy. This combination, which the authors called Mindfulness-Based Cognitive Therapy (MBCT), has been found to reduce the risk of relapse by nearly 50 percent.

Bridges between Science and Consciousness

In 1987, Francisco Varela, a Chilean biologist and neuroscientist; Adam Engle, a lawyer; and His Holiness the Dalai Lama founded the Mind and Life Institute. This institute brought scientists—neuroscientists in particular but also atomic scientists and physicists—together with spiritual practitioners and thinkers to explore the common ground shared by Buddhist, spiritual, and scientific points of view. Francisco Varela observed that Buddhism had been waiting 2,500 years to offer its treasures to the scientific and medical world.

What is the current status of this collaboration between science and meditation? Under the auspices of the Mind and Life Institute, Richard Davidson, a professor of psychology and psychiatry at the University of Wisconsin, Madison, set out to compare the brain activity of nonmeditators with that of monks who were experienced meditators. Davidson asked, "Does something change in the brain of a person who is meditating?" An initial series of tests showed that different parts of the brain are activated, depending on a person's emotional state—happy or unhappy, joyful or sad. When we are happy, joyful, or calm, activity is primarily focused on the left frontal lobe and in the left amygdala. When we are sad, angry, or stressed, activity is focused on certain parts of the right side of the brain, in particular the right amygdala.

This research revealed a second, rather unpleasant, finding. If an individual is born sad or grumpy, he or she keeps this tendency for life. It is a predisposition, possibly genetic. Even if this individual is beautiful and rich, married to an adorable partner, and surrounded by charming children, this negative predisposition will remain. However, when Davidson journeyed to the Himalayas to study the brains of Buddhist monks, what he discovered gave more cause for optimism. Even someone born with a predisposition toward negativity has the potential to change this tendency by practicing meditation. Davidson showed that the more someone meditates, the more the emotional landscape of the brain shifts toward a positive outlook and away from a negative one.

Another study, focusing on the practice of meditating on unconditional love and compassion, was carried out by Davidson, Antoine Lutz, a French neuroscientist based in the United States, and the Buddhist monk Matthieu Ricard. Ricard and seven other experienced meditators agreed to have a series of electrodes attached to the surface of their skulls. Some of these subjects had up to fifty thousand hours of meditation experience—in other words, about five years of meditation. All had practiced a type of meditation known as "nonreferential compassion," or *mikmé nyingjé* in Tibetan. Its aim is to generate a feeling of unconditional loving-kindness and compassion toward all living beings. Antoine Lutz noticed that this meditation had a tendency to make neurons work together. What does that mean? When one is functioning normally, the different regions of one's brain produce waves of different frequencies. When one practices this loving-kindness meditation, however, the neurons tend to vibrate at the same frequency, as if they are in unison. It became clear that through this vibration, separate regions of the brain interconnect, just like workers teaming up to perform a task in synchronicity. Bridges are formed between areas that are not normally accustomed to communicating with each other. It is interesting that this state, which is beneficial for our nervous system, continues beyond the actual meditation session—the brains of the meditators remain in a state of synchronization.

Other studies, undertaken by Sara Lazar, have focused on the plasticity of the brain. At the surface of the brain is a zone called the cortex, which contains our nerve cells. Lazar selected several volunteers who practiced vipassana meditation. Using visual imaging techniques, she noticed that certain zones of the cortex thickened as a result of meditation practice. She also observed that this thickening was greater in those subjects who had meditated for longer.

Thickening of the cortex can have an anti-aging effect, because our cerebral cortex thins as we become older. In people with Alzheimer's disease, the thinning process happens even more quickly. So meditation could perhaps be one way of keeping the mind alert and helping to keep the brain in a youthful state.[2]

We can say that meditation invites connections to be formed on several different levels:

- On a cellular, biological level, meditation facilitates neuronal connections, causing the different neuronal populations in the brain to interrelate.
- On a human level, meditation connects us with the different parts of "me." We realize that we are a thinking "head," working together with a feeling "body."
- On the level of human relationships, when we meditate we realize that we are linked to our fellow human beings, who are just the same as we are.
- On a spiritual level, when we meditate we realize that we are in union with the world around us. We experience the strange truth that this world around us is the same as our inner world, in all its beauty and all its ugliness.
- Beyond all the medical and psychiatric benefits that meditation offers, it also offers a connection to the inexpressible, the invisible, the undecipherable—however we choose to describe it. Spiritual or mystical experiences can arise if we practice meditation, particularly if we do not go looking for them.

What Next?

Where will the dialogue that has been established between science and spirituality take us? I believe we need to see it as an exchange. In the Château de Chambord, built in the sixteenth century by King François I of France, there is a unique staircase, said to have been designed by Leonardo da Vinci, in the form of a double helix. Two people who take the two parts of this staircase at the same time can talk to each other face-to-face, but they will never meet on the same staircase. Such is the dialogue between science and Buddhism. The scientific does not replace the spiritual, and the spiritual does not replace the scientific, but from their collaboration, a fruitful symbiosis is born.

We should beware of the breakneck quest for knowledge at all costs. Even for scientists, a healthy dose of "not-knowing" is recommended, to preserve their ability to be astonished by the world around them. Imagine a hot air balloon filled not with air but with all the knowledge that humans have amassed over time. Everything that the human race has learned is contained inside this balloon, and outside is everything that we do not yet know. We can, of course, fill the balloon with facts, scientific formulae, knowledge of biology, astrology, and so on. But the more the balloon inflates with all this knowledge, the more the unknown—the outside surface of the balloon—grows too. The wisdom contained in the metaphor is that the more we know, the more we realize how much there is still to learn.

To conclude, let us maintain this alliance between science and spirituality. These two paths will perhaps find a meeting point in the search for ultimate truth. As Francisco Varela said, Buddhism has a lot to teach the scientific world. The ancient Buddhist tradition and other forms of meditation contain treasures that are just waiting to be discovered.

4

Training the Mind

The Shamatha Project

Clifford Saron, PhD

In 2007 a team of researchers embarked on the Shamatha Project, the most ambitious and comprehensive study on meditation ever conducted. Using the latest technology, they carried out a wide range of tests on sixty meditators as they took part in three-month retreats in the Rocky Mountains north of Boulder, Colorado. The neuroscientist Clifford Saron led the rigorous effort to examine the effects of meditation on attention, health, empathy, and the emotions. He reveals how this groundbreaking enterprise was planned and implemented, and gives a detailed presentation of the results so far.

Twenty years ago, I was an elderly graduate student with a growing interest in molecular biology. In 1990, my friend and colleague Richard Davidson was scheduled to give a talk at a meeting of the Mind and Life Institute in Dharamsala, India, but he was unable to go. I remember him looking at me with a glint in his eye and asking, "Do you want to go to Dharamsala?" Three weeks later, I found myself giving a presentation to His Holiness the Dalai Lama.[1]

When I arrived in Delhi on the way to Dharamsala, I met a very striking, unusually articulate young man, B. Alan Wallace, now a well-known Buddhist scholar, teacher, and contemplative. Through conversation with Wallace, I learned that for several years he had been thinking that *shamatha* (literally "calm abiding") meditation practice might be amenable to scientific research.[2] Little did I know then that thirteen years later we would be founding the project that I am going to describe here.

In Dharamsala, I ended up sharing a room with Francisco Varela, a neuroscientist, Buddhist practitioner, and a pioneer in the study of self-organizing complex systems. The cofounder of the Mind and Life Institute, he was arguably the intellectual father of the dialogue between scientific and Buddhist contemplative approaches to the study of the mind. Late one night, Varela said to me, "We're old 'EEG-ers.' We should do something—a research project—here in Dharamsala."[3] Even though it was two o'clock in the morning, I was most excited by this proposal and thought he had made a brilliant suggestion that just might change my life. At that time, cognitive neuroscience (the scientific field concerned with elucidating how brain and body create mental life) was still maturing as a field. The Dalai Lama had already expressed an interest in facilitating scientific research regarding Tibetan Buddhist mental training. It seemed a natural extension of the Buddhism-science dialogue for us to embark on a field research project to begin to examine the claims of Tibetan mental training using the nascent tools of cognitive neuroscience. Varela and I put together a team of our colleagues that included Alan Wallace, who was a Tibetan-speaking translator for the Mind and Life meeting, Richard Davidson, Greg Simpson, and José Cabezón. We were able to obtain funds for the project from the Fetzer Institute.

Two years later we embarked on the field study near McLeod Ganj, a small, former British hill station above Dharamsala, where the Dalai Lama lives. Facilitated by the Dalai Lama's Office of Religious and Cultural Affairs, we spoke with advanced Tibetan practitioners who were in retreat on Bhagsu Mountain, above the tiny town of Dharamkot. As we climbed up into the mountains, we followed the goat trails and eventually came to a group of huts. Inside the huts were some extraordinary beings. One monk spoke to us about his meditation practice the way a fine cabinetmaker might speak about his tools. He described how when his mind was dull, he sharpened it; how when it was overexcited, he calmed it; and how when his emotions were turbulent, he treated himself with compassionate regard. This was an extraordinary encounter because we were beginning to think at that point about how we might investigate the effects of such practice, in the form of a specific, collaborative interchange between meditation practitioners and what we as scientists could actually implement in terms of research protocols.

We spent a lot of time thinking about which domains of mental functioning we wanted to investigate in relation to meditation training. We chose four: attention, emotion, language, and visualization. There were many cross-cultural and technical obstacles that limited our ability to collect and analyze all the data as we intended. However, doing this initial project allowed us to think more carefully about how to design and implement some of the experimental tasks that were subsequently included in the Shamatha Project.

Toward the end of our time in Dharamsala, one yogi gave such an extraordinary talk about the nature of compassion that Richard Davidson was moved to make a commitment to introduce compassion to the lexicon of Western academic psychology. We asked this yogi to speak of the relationship between sadness and compassion. He said that while sadness could catalyze the arising of compassion, the two should be considered as separate mindstreams. He explained that one must accept the reality of suffering and try to gain a profound understanding of its causes and conditions. It is ultimately through this understanding that one can most effectively relieve suffering.

Conducting this kind of field research was fraught with a

number of very important cross-cultural issues that suggested to us that it might be more effective to conduct the research in the West.[4] For example, when Varela put on an EEG cap, which uses electrodes to measure electrical activity in the brain, monks from the Institute of Buddhist Dialectics in Dharamsala laughed and said, "How could we be measuring anything to do with the mind by putting a cap on the head? The mind is *here*!"—pointing to their hearts.

Our experiences raised another problem. The extraordinary people we had encountered in this field project might always have been extraordinary. We reasoned that we would actually need to do a longitudinal study to find out how such experience gave rise to a trained mind—that is, we would need to take a group of individuals interested in training their minds with intensive contemplative practice, assess them before, during, and after training, and include similar individuals to test who are not undergoing training to serve as controls, and see what changes ensue. This realization gave rise to the motivation to set up the Shamatha Project.

In 2003, Wallace brought the idea for this project to us at the newly created Center for Mind and Brain at the University of California, Davis. Supported by the Fetzer Institute, the Hershey Family Foundation, and numerous other foundations, funding agencies, and individual donors, we assembled an extraordinary team—a number of dedicated faculty, full-time researchers, post-docs, and graduate students at Davis, supported by a village of consulting scientists and collaborators from around the world.[5]

We set out to look for answers to the following questions:

- Can attention be trained through focused-attention meditation practice?
- Can training in loving-kindness, compassion, and other beneficial aspirations support attention and improve emotion regulation?
- Are improvements in attention related to psychological function?

- What are the subjective, behavioral, neural, and physiological correlates of such training?

The plan was to study a group of thirty meditation practitioners as they took part in a full-time shamatha retreat, practicing for an average of seven hours a day, for three months, under Wallace's guidance. For comparison, we decided to use a control group of thirty meditators with a similar level of experience, because it would have been likely misleading to compare people who wanted to sit for three months in a retreat setting with a random group of adults who did not have any interest in meditation and were not willing to change their lives in any way due to inherent group differences.

To recruit suitable participants we advertised primarily in Buddhist print and Internet publications, and received 142 applications. The applicants were screened to ensure that all of them were physically and psychologically able to take part and had sufficient prior meditation experience. We selected sixty meditators and divided them randomly into two same-size groups, matched for age, sex, education, ethnicity, and meditation experience. We shipped laptop computers loaded up with several computer-based cognitive tasks all over America, Europe, and Mexico in order to gather some behavioral data from our subjects before they even knew whether they would be part of the initial retreat group or the control group.

While the first group began their three-month retreat, the thirty in the control group were flown to the retreat center, where they underwent the same tests as the retreat group at roughly the same time, but without embarking on the same intensive meditation practice. Three months after the first retreat had finished, the control group took part in the same three-month retreat program, again taught by Alan Wallace. Our emphasis was not so much on what actually happens while you are meditating but what happens because you have dedicated time to meditation—in other words, we were looking for trait changes (what you *do* differently *because* you have meditated). We tested the control group in the same way as we did the participants in retreat, and followed up both groups at five and sixteen months after each retreat.

This format enabled us to use the control group in two ways: First, we could compare their results with those of the retreatants who were meditating full-time. Second, we were able to use the control group's results when they were not in retreat as an extensive baseline to compare with their own results when they subsequently went into retreat. We had very committed participants across a broad age range, from twenty-one to seventy. Virtually everyone stayed for the full length of their retreat, and every one of the control subjects made the three six-day trips to be tested. We even had very good compliance for follow-up testing.

This entire study was conducted in the spring and fall of 2007 at Shambhala Mountain Center in the Rocky Mountains northeast of Boulder, Colorado. It was certainly an interesting environment for a scientific study. We were able to secure for six months a lodge that had never really been used before. It had a meditation hall and, on the floor below, a dormitory room that we thought would make a superb field laboratory space. So we took out the beds and built two side-by-side university-grade psychophysiology labs, each complete with a testing room and an equipment control room. In the testing room, participants could undergo a variety of attention- and emotion-related experiments. In one instance, we used a video camera concealed by a speaker so that we could unobtrusively record participants' facial expressions. From the control room we recorded EEG signals and measures of autonomic nervous system physiology such as heart rate, blood pressure, respiration, and emotional sweating. We also tested the startle response by presenting a loud noise while people were viewing photographs selected to elicit positive or negative emotional experiences. Emotional states change the startle response, so we could examine the time course and intensity of emotion elicited by specific images, as a function of training. This was one way to index the recovery time after an emotional provocation. We also built a blood lab in an adjacent room so that we could prepare samples for biochemical analysis. At the end we tore it all apart. It was like a "sand mandala" laboratory.[6]

During the retreats, Wallace taught two complementary forms of meditation practice for focusing the mind and opening the heart. The first element was shamatha meditation using several different techniques: "mindfulness of breathing in three phases," based on the Theravada Buddhist tradition; "settling the mind in its natural state," also known as observing the mind, as taught in the Dzogchen tradition of shamatha, which in scientific parlance is called observing mental events; and awareness of awareness, also known as shamatha without an object, as taught in the Dzogchen tradition of shamatha. Wallace also taught the practices of the Four Immeasurables (loving-kindness, compassion, empathetic joy, and equanimity) as guided meditations, which the retreatants included in their individual practice.[7]

Hypotheses, Experiments, and Results

Our expectations from this project in essence can be boiled down to four domains of change: (1) an improved ability to focus; (2) increased access to experience, no matter what it feels like; (3) faster recovery from provocation; and (4) diminution of destructive tendencies.

We had three or four years of discussions while we were trying to raise the money to begin the project, so we had a lot of time to think about the various ways in which we could set up experiments to test these predictions. Although we have some interest in examining what goes on physiologically during meditation, we were primarily interested in keeping careful track of how much and what type of meditation people were practicing, so we could relate this information to changes in their mood states, significant emotional events, and experimental data. We had participants fill out daily experience questionnaires every day. We used the tools of modern social psychology and psychometrics, which included personality trait questionnaires and new surveys regarding mindfulness, well-being, and self-compassion developed as part of the growth of this field. We also performed structured interviews, because we knew that no questionnaire could get at the nature of someone's individual experience and adequately capture the uniqueness of this person's goals, challenges, and insights. If you have a record of how the world unfolds for someone, it can be coded, rigorously and quantitatively. (The analysis of the structured interviews is ongoing, spearheaded by Baljinder Sahdra of the University of Western Sydney and Susan Bauer-Wu at the University of Virginia.)

We also had laboratory-based emotion-related tasks, emotion-interaction tasks, and attention-related tasks. All told, we conducted fifteen computer-based experiments.[8]

Self-Reported Psychological Changes

The daily mood questionnaire that we gave people asked them to rate, on a scale of 1 to 7, forty-two words describing positive and negative moods. Both the retreatants and the control participants filled out these questionnaires every day, over the course of the three-month retreat. We examined how different words were rated together and performed a statistical analysis that clustered some of the words into different "factors" such as ill-being and well-being. When we averaged the ratings from all the questionnaires, the level of the well-being factor in the control group stayed relatively flat over the three months, but with ups and downs, while for the retreat group it slowly increased. When the control participants entered their own retreat, they showed the same gentle rise over three months. When we share the results of our experiments, some people tend to respond, "Oh, it's a meditation retreat. Isn't that just like a vacation?" Of course, no one who has ever participated in a retreat would attribute his growth in well-being over time just to external circumstances, and a retreat can often be a complex, challenging period of time. In fact, it is the steady rate of growth of well-being over time that argues against the notion that any positive changes are easily attributable to the "vacation effect." Instead, the gradual growth of well-being, which was replicated in the second retreat, suggests that a fundamental internal shift is resulting from the meditation training and in learning to deal with and accept the conditions of one's mind.

In a 2011 paper whose lead author was Baljinder Sahdra we describe how we combined the information in the many other questionnaires into one construct that we called "adaptive functioning." An increase in adaptive functioning means there has been an increase in well-being, mindfulness, empathy, and ego resiliency and a decrease in depression, anxiety, neuroticism, and difficulties in emotion regulation.[9] Over the three-month period there was no difference on these measures within the control group. The retreat group, however, showed a significant increase in adaptive functioning, and it was sustained when tested five months later. When members of the control group themselves became retreatants, they showed the exact same pattern.[10]

We were aware that some participants in our study might be showing some "response bias"—the tendency to respond as they feel they *should*, to try to give answers they think researchers want to hear. The question then arises of what other changes we found, and whether the results from our other experiments or measures support the findings from these questionnaires.

Cortisol and Mindfulness

An important component of our research study included the investigation of observable biological changes that occurred as a result of intensive meditation training. The body and mind are intimately connected, and so in the spirit of being as comprehensive as possible, we chose to index biological markers, in addition to experimental tasks, in order to obtain more objective measures, in addition to self-reports, that could substantiate our claims.

Cortisol is a stress-related hormone with widespread physiological effects that help marshal the body's resources in response to acute stress, but whose consequences are harmful if it is chronically oversecreted. One of our hypotheses was that the process of worrying and ruminating over past or future events may prolong cortisol release, which in turn may contribute to creating predisease pathways and adversely affect physical health. Specifically, we were interested in investigating the link between self-reported mindfulness and cortisol. To do this, we measured both self-reported mindfulness and afternoon and evening, or "P.M.," cortisol levels (the latter being the combined values of two hours after lunch and just before bedtime) near the beginning and end of the three-month meditation retreat. We found that although mindfulness increased from pre- to post-retreat, cortisol did not significantly change after the retreat, which was contrary to our predictions. However, this was just a "first cut" picture of the data. With further analysis we found an interesting pattern of findings more in line with our predictions.[11]

First, we found that mindfulness was inversely related to P.M. cortisol at both pre-retreat and post-retreat, even when accounting for age and body mass index. Then we found that changes in mindfulness between pre- and post-retreat were associated with changes in P.M. cortisol (from pre- to post-retreat). Indeed, larger increases in mindfulness were associated with decreases in P.M. cortisol, while smaller increases (or slight decreases) in mindfulness, as assessed by three facets of mindfulness reflected in the training (mindful observing, mindful acting, and mindful nonreacting), were associated with an increase in P.M. cortisol).

These findings are illuminating, since no overall change in P.M. cortisol was observed in the study until we examined results in terms of individual differences in change in mindfulness as self-reported by means of the questionnaire. However, it will be important to see if these findings can be replicated in a larger cohort and with more rigorous control-group conditions, such as a group of individuals doing a different kind of training.

Telomerase and Stress Reduction

Telomerase is an enzyme that is crucial to the process of cell division. Cells in the body undergo a division process known as mitosis in order to pass on genetic material from one generation of cells to the next. During mitosis, the parent cell first copies its DNA and then divides into two daughter cells, and passes on a copy of each of its two chromosomes, the structures that carry genetic information, to each daughter cell. The ends of these chromosomes are capped by repeating DNA sequences, known as telomeres, that regulate the integrity of genetic transmission. However, the telomeres are not fully copied each time cells divide and they grow shorter with each subsequent cell division. When telomeres grow too short, cells cannot divide. This is where telomerase comes in: it restores the length of telomeres. Our collaborator Elizabeth Blackburn and her colleagues Carolyn W. Greider and Jack W. Szostak won the 2009 Nobel Prize in Physiology or Medicine for their discovery of telomeres and telomerase. Interesting to note, the length of telomeres predicts longevity. A study done by our collaborator Elissa Epel and her research group at the University of California, San Francisco, Medical Center on men with heart disease showed that if a man's telomeres shortened over a two-and-a-half-year period, there was a 50 percent chance he would be dead within ten years. If his telomeres did not get shorter in that two-and-a-half-year period, there was an 87 percent chance he would still be alive after ten years. So telomeres are central to longevity.[12]

Telomerase levels may change the effective shortening of your telomeres over time. Although a complex story, it appears that telomerase levels can be increased by well-being and decreased by stress. A study by Elissa Epel and her colleagues demonstrated that telomerase is suppressed in mothers who have high perceived levels of stress while they are caring for children with autism or life-threatening illnesses.[13] Other studies have shown that telomerase levels can also be increased. A study by Dean Ornish and his colleagues showed that with a strict diet, exercise, a *little* meditation, and a healthy lifestyle, telomerase levels go up.[14] This would lead us to predict the same kind of results from the Shamatha Project. In our study Tonya Jacobs, Elissa Epel, and colleagues measured telomerase levels and found that the control group had 30 percent less telomerase than the retreat group at the end of the first three-month retreat, which is the same degree of change that was seen in the study by Ornish.[15] Furthermore, these telomerase levels were related to individual differences in psychological change over the course of the retreat, providing a strong link between biological changes and psychological function.

It is important to note that stress itself is not necessarily a bad thing, but chronic stress, a condition that limits your ability to deal with challenges, can be a huge problem. Organisms are always working toward maintaining internal stability through processes known as homeostasis and allostasis. Homeostasis refers to the body's return to balance via physiological regulation of such things as blood pressure, blood glucose, temperature, and acidity. In contrast, allostasis refers to the ability of an organism to achieve net internal stability by remaining more dynamic and variable from moment to moment. Allostasis is, in a sense, your ability, in real time, to meet challenges.

One of the hypotheses regarding the benefits of meditation practice is that meditation can, over time, enhance your ability to meet challenges and mobilize your resources. The idea is that you can constantly, at some level, not take it all so seriously—because you have become a little less identified with the "I" that you think is "you." The basic premise is that meditative practices may increase a construct called "mindfulness," and our research team and other colleagues have begun a discussion of the multiple ways in which this can be conceptualized.[16] If you have increases in mindfulness and a sense of direction and purpose in your life, it may increase your stress resilience and your capacity to meet challenges, and decrease your stress vulnerability. Stress vulnerability is highly related to neuroticism—our tendency to make mountains out of molehills. Stress resilience, however, can be defined as having a sense of mastery—also called perceived control—over the conditions of our lives.

There are many different schools of thought on how to define and measure mindfulness.[17] One current methodology used by psychologists is via questionnaires.[18] Questionnaires allow us to index a variety of other psychological measures, such as "neuroticism," "perceived control," and "purpose in life." We tracked changes in self-reported psychological measures over a three-month period and found that an increase in "mindfulness" was significantly greater for the retreat participants than for the control group. We also found increases in measures of "purpose in life" and "perceived control" for the retreatants, and a decrease in "neuroticism."[19]

In addition, we found a significant correlation between the amount of telomerase activity (measured from a type of circulating white blood cells known as monocytes) measured at the end of the first retreat and the change in "perceived control" for retreat participants—but not for the control group. In the retreat participants, higher levels of telomerase measured at the end of the retreat were associated with increases in "perceived control" and "purpose in life" and a decrease in "neuroticism" across the span of the retreat.

The telomerase findings weaken the argument that positive changes observed via reports in questionnaires are due to participants' response bias. Furthermore, these findings are compelling because they provide us with a link between biomarkers and self-reported psychological changes. I am not suggesting that meditation will make you live a longer life. I am not saying that meditation alone raises your telomerase levels or results in longer telomeres. That claim will be tested in future work. But this kind of finding will motivate that work. It does look as though activities that foster meaningful positive psychological change, such as meditation, positively impact cellular aging.

Attention and Perception

The people who took part in these three-month retreats with Alan Wallace were very dedicated to their practice. Some of them were able and willing to meditate for up to twelve hours a day. One of the core claims about this practice is that returning your mind again and again to an object of focus, while simultaneously monitoring the quality of your attention on that object, should result in improvements in sustained attention that generalize to other tasks in daily life.

How do you measure improved sustained attention? Most of the tasks that currently exist are designed to try to diagnose individuals with attention deficit disorder, and there has been remarkably little research on the training of attention. From World War II onward, researchers investigating whether radar operators could stay in front of their consoles for hour after hour have characterized improving attention through training as a hopelessly difficult task. They thought that one could only really pay attention for a few minutes before attention levels inevitably started to drop.

To put the claim that attention cannot be maintained to the test, Katherine MacLean devised a task for measuring attention called the continuous performance task for target detection (CPT).[20] In this test, sustained attention was defined as the ability to quickly perceive minuscule differences between the lengths of two lines throughout the course of the experiment.

Before the full thirty-minute task begins, we determine each individual's unique "perceptual threshold"—that is, the point at which an individual is barely able to reliably discriminate between two very similar stimuli. To determine this perceptual threshold, we present participants with lines of varying length, with one line appearing on the screen in front of them about every two seconds. Each line is presented briefly (about one-tenth of a second). Most of the time the line is "long" (about 5 centimeters). Sometimes the line is a bit shorter. The subject's task is to press a button when he or she spots the short line.

Shortly after participants first begin the task, we present the short line very close in length to the long line, causing them to make many errors—that is, they no longer notice the short line and fail to press the button in response to the target. At this point, we start making the line shorter again. Once the participant can differentiate short from long lines reliably, then we make the shorter lines longer again until they more closely resemble the longer lines. We do this again and again until we converge on each individual's perceptual threshold. After the subjects reach about 75 percent accuracy to detect a given "short line" length (which takes about ten minutes), the full task begins using long and short lines that do not change in length during the experiment.

Both the retreat and control groups performed this perceptual and button-pushing task about every two seconds for thirty-two minutes without a break. They were asked to press a button only when they saw the short line, which occurred in about one in ten presented lines. The two groups were both measured for their performance in this task pre-retreat. At this point there was no difference between the two groups. After five weeks of meditation, however, the retreat group was significantly better able than the control group to perceive a shorter line closer in length to the long line. They had increased vividness of perception, which was sustained at the end of the retreat and five months later at follow-up. When the control group went into retreat, by the midpoint of their retreat they showed the same pattern as the first retreat group, and this improvement was sustained at their five-month follow-up, provided that the control group members had continued to meditate each day (which was also true for the first retreat group).

Results from the control group and pre-retreat data showed that when you are not meditating in retreat, your performance declines over time in this task, as was expected. This is why we do not have the same person watching an X-ray screening machine at the airport all day long. However, by the midpoint of the retreat, and at the end, the meditators had better sustained ability to detect this target. Given the change in perceptual threshold, our hypothesis is that the ability to continue to detect slight differences—two lines that are almost the same length—is actually related to changes in perception. This is an important point. It is not so much that attention per se improved but that the task actually got easier for the meditators because they were able to perceive the signal more easily, because their threshold to see small visual differences improved.

In addition to behavioral measures, we looked at brain activity in order to compare the brain response to the long line (the non-target) and the short line (the target). In the second retreat, the stimuli in this experiment did not change from the beginning to the end of the retreat. At the beginning of the retreat, brain responses to short and long lines (which look very similar) did not differ. At the end of the retreat, the target short line elicited a larger brain response, indicating increased perceptual processing of the target item, and the non-target (the long line that subjects did not respond to) elicited a smaller brain response, indicating decreased perceptual processing of the non-target. That means the meditators' brains had become, in effect, optimized to generate a larger signal from a tiny perceptual difference.[21]

In looking closely at the brain activity, we discovered another interesting relationship between the neural patterns we observed before, during, and after the task, and the subsequent behavioral responses made by the participants. We noticed a link between decreased alpha brain waves (defined here as EEG power in the frequency range of 8 to 12 hertz) and sustained attention performance. When you have more alpha-wave activity in a particular brain region, there is often relatively less cortical activation in that region. For instance, when you close your eyes, you have less visual activity and, typically, a very large increase in alpha EEG activity recordable over the visual cortex (primarily the posterior or occipital and parietal brain regions). Individuals who participated in a three-month retreat demonstrated decreased alpha levels in the occipito-parietal region of the cortex immediately prior to the perception of a stimulus.

In addition, the magnitude of the decrease in alpha-wave activity that occurred just prior to the appearance of each long or short line predicted how well individuals maintained their vigilance to detect the short lines. Individuals who did not show much change from pre- to post-retreat in their alpha-wave activity before the stimulus was presented also did not show much improvement in their performance of the task. In contrast, individuals who showed a large decrease in the alpha-wave levels pre-stimulus demonstrated improved performance in the task. Thus, there is an association between one's brain state as inferred from the EEG (akin to being better prepared to perceive) and one's actual performance.

Response Inhibition

In a related task, the response inhibition task (RIT), instead of pressing the button when presented with the short line, participants were asked to press the button in response to *all* the long lines, which appear 90 percent of the time, and to *withhold* their response to the short lines. The short lines were still targets, but now a response to a target meant to *stop* the habitual, frequent motor response of pushing the button. Just as with the CPT, there was a performance decline over time for all participants when not in retreat. However, when individuals participated in the meditation retreats, midway through the retreat they began showing less of a decline in their performance, and by the end of the three months the performance decline decreased even more.[22]

Performance in this task was not related to perceptual threshold. Improved stability on this task seemed to be related, rather, to improvements in an absolutely critical cognitive skill: executive control. "Executive control" is the large umbrella term for all the processes in the brain that allow you to maintain goals and to inhibit inappropriate responses. Much of Buddhist practice has to do with exercising very high levels of executive control. It was interesting that younger participants—those under fifty—who did not meditate that much in their outside lives demonstrated greater improvement in this task than older participants.

Through complex statistical modeling procedures, we found that improvements in response inhibition pre- to mid-retreat actually predicted individuals' improvements in psychological adaptive functioning pre- to post-retreat. The importance and beauty of this finding was its ability to connect a low-level, boring, response-inhibition experiment to participants' self-reported experience, as revealed in the questionnaires. In Buddhist teachings, individuals are encouraged to cultivate the ability to withhold "knee-jerk" responses in emotionally charged situations or relationships, and instead act from a more grounded and wise place.

Emotions

In addition to our interests in indexing the biological, neural, and behavioral changes that result from participating in an intensive meditation retreat, we were also interested in emotion. Specifically, we were interested in investigating whether people's emotional responses changed during the course of the retreat and, perhaps even more important, whether individuals had greater insight into their emotional responses as a result of the training.

To investigate, we set out to create a situation in which individuals were emotionally provoked by film clips depicting scenes of human suffering. Participants' facial expressions were recorded unobtrusively while they were watching the films. In addition, we obtained self-report measures by asking participants to indicate the type and intensity of emotions they felt during the film. Immediately after the film ended, we asked them about their emotions and we cued recall of the film by presenting a kind of storyboard of the clip with frames that depicted film content every two seconds.

We then used a system called the Facial Action Coding System (FACS), developed by Paul Ekman and Walter Friesen, that describes forty-six separate facial muscle groups that can be visibly coded from video records.[23] Two graduate students, Brandon King and Anthony Zanesco, led by the emotion researcher and master FACS teacher Erika Rosenberg coded our video records frame by frame in order to identify precisely the timing and intensity of the movements of facial muscles, described as "action units." From these measurements of facial movement, we obtained a full database of facial behavior over time. By grouping the close occurrence of different action units together and using an emotional facial expression dictionary, we can infer the emotion someone was expressing at a particular moment in time in response to the film clips.

This coding of facial expressions is remarkably labor-intensive. It takes roughly two and a half hours to code one minute of facial behavior, so coding responses to a single two-minute film clip is more than a good day's work. This facial coding was performed on twenty-nine retreatants and twenty-nine controls at the beginning and end of the first retreat.

One of the film clips that we showed to participants at the end of the retreat period was from *Fahrenheit 9/11*. The clip begins by showing scenes of daily life in Iraq prior to the war, such as kids playing in the streets and citizens frequenting restaurants. Next, the clip suddenly moves to scenes of bombing and missile strikes. It then alternates between soldiers talking about how they get pumped up to go into battle and scenes of war victims suffering. Eventually, other soldiers begin to reflect on the real consequences of their actions, stating that "this ain't no video game," and more scenes of war victims are shown.

We found that after three months of meditation training, more retreatants showed expressions of sadness than the control participants, suggesting that there may be an increased level of engagement and sympathy with the suffering of others after intensive meditation practice. In support of this interpretation are two other findings: retreat participants' self-reported sympathy ratings were positively related to the number of sadness behaviors expressed over the course of the film, and the retreatants also expressed *fewer* rejection emotions (a cluster of contempt, disgust, and anger emotions) than the control group.

We had predicted that we would observe less rejection of graphic suffering in the meditators than in the control group. And this is what in fact occurred. The reason for our prediction rested on the fact that the ability to learn how to encounter suffering directly, with less aversion in doing so, is part of Buddhist training. In contrast, the control group's aversion may have been growing throughout the clip, for they actually showed increasing rejection emotions across the duration of the film clip.[24]

Conclusions

The various experiments under the larger umbrella of our longitudinal study have certainly illuminated our understanding of a wide range of emotional and behavioral changes that result from participating in an intensive meditation training. First, our results demonstrated that retreatants' daily reports of mood and psychological traits are consistent with improved well-being. One interesting finding was that these changes were related to increased levels of telomerase, an enzyme that plays a crucial role in protecting cells from premature aging. We also discovered that retreatants demonstrated improvements in their visual perception and vigilance in the sustained-attention task, and these improvements were related to threshold changes. Brain responses that we measured demonstrated improved discrimination between small physical differences in stimuli after training, and these responses were related to pre-stimulus activation differences in the brain. We also noted that improvements in response inhibition occurred and that these improvements actually predicted improved adaptive psychological functioning. Self-reports in response to emotional provocation in film tasks differed between retreat and control groups. In addition, retreatants were more likely to show expressions of sadness and showed fewer expressions of rejection emotions than did the control participants, demonstrating, after intensive meditation practice, increased engagement and sympathy with the observable suffering of others.

We face many issues as we attempt to perform rigorous research in this field. For example, what kinds of changes result simply from committing time to sitting—changing your life in all of the ways that you do when you commit to a contemplative practice? It's what I call the "tuches effect."[25] Beyond anything to do with your philosophy, or your understanding of dharma, or the specific meditation instructions you follow, if you close your eyes for six hours a day—or keep them open softly with no particular focus—your visual system will change. You may begin to learn new behavioral habits that ramify into daily life in untold ways. Conversely, your worldview may have an enormous impact on the effects of any practice that you do. So we have worldview, the social support of joining a group retreat, and neuroplastic reorganization because of behavioral change. What, exactly, is the intervention? It is, in toto, much more than following specific meditation instructions. Thus, the results of our experiments have unearthed as many questions as they have answered, as is often the case with scientific research.

That being said, the Shamatha Project is truly a groundbreaking study. It is the first longitudinal study of its kind with as deeply matched a randomized wait list control group and as comprehensive a set of measures.[26] Another thing that makes the Shamatha Project unique is the way it draws on various methods of analysis from diverse fields ranging from cognitive neuroscience to biology to social psychology and anthropology.

As we carry on with our analyses on this complex data set with new support from a large grant from the John Templeton Foundation,[27] and indeed as we continue to investigate important questions within the field of contemplative science as a whole, we must bear in mind the multidimensional nature of something so intricate as the nature of the human mind and self-directed growth and transformation. The field faces numerous challenges, but with the scientific methods at our disposal and with an honest acknowledgment not only of the strengths but also of the limitations of these investigative methodologies, we are poised to continue scientifically investigating Buddhist mental training and what such training means for our study participants with potentially broad beneficial application.[28]

5

Meditation and Emotion

Erika Rosenberg, PhD

Our emotions have a powerful influence on our state of mind, our happiness, and even our health, but do we have any control over them? Erika Rosenberg, who is a consulting scientist at the Center for Mind and Brain at the University of California, Davis, is a leading expert in the study of emotions and a meditation teacher. She takes us on a step-by-step journey through the emotional process, and explains what can happen when you add a little meditation into the mix.

As a scientist I have been studying emotions for over twenty years. During that time, I have also been practicing meditation and teaching it to others. In both of these enterprises, I have focused in particular on emotions, because I have found that they play a profound role in my life, and I know that they can be the source of both great joy and suffering. For many years, these two lines of work were independent, but in the last decade they have come together. Now I am committed to bringing science and meditation instruction together, in order to benefit people. I am going to explore here how this dual perspective has affected my understanding of emotion, both as a researcher and as a meditation teacher.

When the ways science and meditation come together and how the practical benefits of these two fields overlap are discussed, it is often pointed out that meditation and science share an approach. I would like to point out another similarity, which is that science and meditation are both empirical processes—they are rooted in observation. As a scientist, you might have notions about how things work, but you will consult the outside world, observe factors such as behavior, bodily function, weather patterns, and so on, and see whether these observations, when obtained systematically and analyzed, correspond with your own notions of how the world works. If they do not, you modify your view. That is one of the ways in which science differs from philosophy. Science is more about observation than logic. Perhaps it should be more about logic at times, but it is really about whether your views or thoughts are consistent with what you find when you study these ideas in the world.

Meditation is also about observation, but it is an inner inquiry. Our journey as meditators is all about examining the mind, so we ask questions about how our own minds work, and we learn that we should not necessarily believe our thoughts. We are studying and gaining increased objectivity in relation to our own thoughts, emotions, and experiences. The two might be very different on the surface, but meditation and science are both empirical processes, and they can inform each other.

Emotions arise in response to things that matter to us. We do not have emotional responses to things that do not matter. Events in the world, thoughts, ideas, memories, things that stimulate our senses but also have some meaning to our physical safety, our goals in life, our well-being—these are the events to which we respond emotionally. When we have these responses, they are very powerful. Our heart might start racing, our skin will get moist, we might feel that we have to move. This is why we pay so much attention to our emotions, and why they can be the source of so much joy and suffering in our lives. They can overwhelm us.

When considering the powerful effect that emotions have on our bodies and on our thoughts and minds, we often have the feeling that they happen *to* us. We think, *Oh! All of a sudden I was angry. All of a sudden I was afraid. I don't know where that came from.* My mentor Paul Ekman, a leading expert in the study of facial expressions of emotion, has used the word "unbidden" for this feeling. It seems to us that emotions simply happen, and for some reason that creates a sense that they are outside us. But that is not the case. They are products of our own minds; they emerge from our own thoughts. Emotions arise as a function of how we see the world, but the fact remains that they are really powerful, and they can overtake our bodies.

Another thing that is very important to remember is that an emotional reaction is *fast*. When we study people's emotional reactions in laboratories, we observe that emotions are very brief. Sometimes they last a matter of seconds. When I say this to people, they reply, "But I've been miserable for a whole day," or, "I've been sad for hours." Usually what is happening in such cases is that there is a revisiting of the emotions, or repeated occurrences of the same type of emotion. If we have been sad, we keep thinking about what makes us sad. The sadness itself becomes the basis for more sadness, and there is a recurring cycle. We get sad over and over again. For any given emotion, the major changes that occur in our bodies when we encounter something that is significant to us move through us quickly and then they go. But they persist and seem long-lasting if we get into a recurring cycle.

The reason why emotions happen in this way is related to their evolutionary origins. According to evolutionary biology and evolutionary psychology, emotions evolve for their ability to help us respond quickly to certain critical situations in the environment. This is important in helping us to understand how emotions affect us so potently. For example, if in our ancestral past, I had been picking berries and suddenly a beast had appeared in front of me on the trail, it would have been adaptive for me to be able to move and get out of the way very quickly. If I had to sit there and think, *Hmm, perhaps this is a dangerous situation, maybe I should move*, by the time I got to the end of that thought I might possibly be dead.

This is an example from human evolution, but we can go even further back, because we know that nonhuman, nonprimate animals also have emotions. Creatures who had this ability to generate a bodily response that motivated movement really quickly, without much thought, could respond more quickly and efficiently to critical situations in the environment than creatures who lacked it. That is the standard evolutionary account for emotion. I will leave it to you to reflect on whether that explanation works for all kinds of emotions, but it certainly works for negative emotions such as fear.

This account explains why certain changes happen all of a sudden: the heart rate increases, the breathing speeds up, and the heart pumps blood to the skeletal muscles so that you can move and get away from the source of danger. Of course, we do not encounter situations like that very often in our lives these days, but sometimes we do. You could be driving down a highway and all of a sudden a car pulls in front of you, and you have to step on the brake very quickly in order to save your life. If you had to sit and do a rational analysis at that particular moment, the outcome would not be very positive.

Thus, there are situations in which a quick response is very helpful. But there are many other situations in which our ancestral past hijacks our well-being. We do not need to have that kind of response when we are anticipating encountering a difficult situation at work, for example. A little bit of anxiety might help us to prepare, but it can build up in a way that paralyzes us. That is why it is so important to understand how emotions work, and to learn how to work with them. If we understand that they are brief, even though they create powerful changes, we can learn to ride them out.

It is also important to understand that emotions themselves, in terms of the changes that happen when we experience them, are neither good nor bad. Some emotions feel good and others do not feel good, but the actual "good" or "bad," the positive or negative, is really more a function of what ends up coming out of the situation. Let's say that someone does something that insults you, and you start feeling the energy of anger coming up in your body. If you ride that anger out, just breathe and let it go, it will pass. But if, as soon as the anger comes up, you say something nasty back to the person who has insulted you, that is the destructive part. What counts is the behavior that the emotion motivates.

Emotions themselves are not suffering. Just as thoughts happen, emotions just happen. We might, with inner work and a lot of practice, start changing the way we see situations, which will change the kinds of emotions we have, but we are still going to have emotions. The point of meditation is not to eliminate emotions. It is to learn how to accommodate them skillfully and with compassion for oneself and others. I have talked to people who have been practicing meditation for thirty-five years in a monastic tradition, and guess what—they still have emotions! Suffering results from the behavior motivated by the emotion—whether you say something you will later regret, or you do something that is ultimately going to be destructive for you, like drinking too much.

Suffering can also result from the way we relate to our emotions. Say you have been waiting for ages in a long line at the supermarket and all of a sudden someone rudely pushes in front of you. When you finally leave the store you are furious, because what that person did was not fair. But what do you do next? Hours later, are you still thinking about that clever thing you could have said in order to get back at the queue-jumper? We can go on and on like this, and most of the situations in which we do this in our lives are very trivial. Maybe someone made an obscene hand gesture at you while you were waiting in traffic, and you keep stewing about it. After a while, you realize you have wasted about two hours of your day thinking about this trivial event. That's suffering! Sometimes, it is true, genuinely dramatic, traumatic things happen in our lives. But a lot of the suffering that creates the physiological effects of stress that have a negative impact on our mental and physical health is just about grasping at and revisiting trivial unpleasant events.

Suffering also results from emotions about emotions. Just as we tend to keep revisiting the sadness when we are sad, we do the same with anxiety. Let's say we have a big project due, a big performance we have to give, or an hour in which to finish an exam. We start thinking about it and we get anxious, and then what happens is what I call "emotion about emotion," or "affect about affect." We feel anxiety about the fact that we are anxious. This happens to people who have trouble sleeping at night. They might already feel a little agitated, and then they start thinking, *Oh no, what if I can't fall asleep*? That creates more anxiety, and they think, *What if it gets to two o'clock and I still can't fall asleep*? They keep building it up and building it up. That is another kind of suffering that emotions can create.

I would like to present a view of emotion that I believe helps us to understand not just how emotions work, but also the opportunities for change and the kinds of qualities and skills that we can cultivate through meditative practice. This is a view of emotion as a process, an idea that will not be new for anyone with a background in psychology. Elements of this view draw on the appraisal theorists, such as Richard Lazarus, and on evolutionary theorists as well. According to this view, emotions always start with something that we might call an antecedent event. The emotion has not actually started yet, but there has to be something in the world, either in your mind or something as simple as stepping in something nasty on the sidewalk, that you look at and you evaluate. It could be a memory, it could be seeing your friend's face, or seeing the dog poop on the sidewalk—that is the antecedent event. You evaluate what this means to you, and this is what we call appraisal.

It is very important to point out that this appraisal, this evaluation of the significance of an event—whatever it might be—is often not conscious. Most of the time, especially if we consider the survival value of having emotions, it is probably going to be very quick and very automatic. Sometimes the appraisal is conscious, but often it is not, and there is a very quick process of evaluation. If this event is meaningful to the person concerned, then an emotion will ensue. If the event is not meaningful, it will not generate an emotion. For example, if you are walking down the street and you suddenly see someone who is meaningful to you, you think: *Oh, there's Sara. I haven't seen her in so long.* Then an emotion comes.

Once an emotion is generated, all kinds of things happen, and this is the stage that we call emotional response. There is a physiological response from the autonomic nervous system—the branch of the nervous system that controls all the processes that are usually self-governing and occur without conscious control, such as changes in heart rate, skin conductance, and secretion of the glands. These are all activated. Behavioral tendencies are activated—whether you want to move toward or away from something, for example. Thoughts, too, are activated. The cognition component is a network of memories and associations, maybe from the last time you saw Sara, or the last time you were in a similar kind of feeling state. There are often, but not always, behavioral expressive elements, such as facial expression changes. There could be vocal expression changes as well, because the vocal cords are innervated by the autonomic nervous system, and during emotional arousal the pitch of the voice goes up. Also important are experiential changes, and by that I mean the quality of what it feels like to be happy or sad, guilty, jealous, or amused. All of this happens really, really fast.

Now let us turn to meditation. If you cultivate certain qualities through meditation—let's say you have been working with relaxation, or just simple stability and calmness—there are suddenly opportunities to intervene at each stage of the emotional process. Sara Lazar's research on stress showed that there was a change in the size of the amygdala that was not reversed when the meditators went back to the same stressful work environment and the same stressful lives. This implies that it is not the situation that counts, but how you evaluate it.[1] The antecedent event is the stimulus, but you have flexibility in how you respond to it. This is where the freedom lies.

You are not bound to a reflex, like when someone hits the patellar tendon of your knee with a hammer and you can't prevent your knee from jerking. Any situation presents an infinite amount of flexibility, so this is one place where there is a huge opportunity for change.

If you have been doing basic *shamatha* practice, stabilizing the mind and cultivating a quality of calm, one thing that happens fairly quickly is that you just *are* calmer; and if you create more calmness in your body, you can use this as an antidote if something agitates you. You can calm yourself down. That is one of the gifts of meditative practice. You know how to do it, and you can apply it when you need to. But what about trait changes? Can you make yourself a calmer person? If you are a calmer person, presumably you will be less reactive. When I teach meditation, I often use the age-old metaphor of water. If the water in a glass is agitated and there is any sediment or silt in it, you will not be able to see through the water. If you stop stirring a glass of water, the sediment will settle and you will be left with this clear space. If you think of that clear space as a metaphor for mind, you are now able to see better.

What I love about the glass-of-water metaphor is that when the dirt is settled in the water, although the water is clear, you can still see the stuff that is in the sediment. That is where the mindfulness comes in handy, because you can notice what is in your mind. If you can see your habitual tendencies that might lead you to think that the world is out to get you, or that you are always going to get the short end of the stick, you can decide, *Well, that's one way of thinking that I follow a lot of the time, but I don't have to think like that. Look at all this clear, open space. My mind can go somewhere else.* Meditation can therefore have a huge impact on the appraisal stage of the process, which is what drives the emotion.

The quality of the appraisal determines what kind of emotion results. If you see a situation as one of threat to your physical safety and your goals, which might mean you do not get what you want, it can lead to anxiety or fear. If someone has thwarted you or insulted you, it usually leads to anger. If there is a situation of loss, it brings sadness. But it is all about how you see the situation. We know that two people can go into the same situation and have a very different emotional response to it.

You may not be able to control exactly what happens to you in the world, but you can control how you respond to it, and that is where freedom lies. Thus, there is a lot of opportunity for change at the appraisal stage. If you have cultivated a sense of calm, you also have the opportunity to influence how the emotional response stage goes. You cannot necessarily prevent it from happening, but if you have cultivated a calmer foundation—this is empirically testable and we have the data to look at this—you may not have as big a reaction and you may recover more quickly.

Once the emotional response has happened, if you let that energy move through and realize that you do not have to identify with it or grasp it, you can simply feel those energetic changes and they will subside. The other response you can have when this happens is to get very upset, scared, or angry about the fact that you have an emotion, and to keep feeding it. If you are calm, if the mind is clear, and if you have cultivated mindfulness, you can make more choices about what you can do once this emotion has arisen. Perhaps most important, you can make choices with your eyes open about how you act. I am not coming from a scientific perspective here; I am coming from the experiential data as a meditation practitioner. The whole process slows down.

If you become familiar with the changes that happen in your body, you can catch an emotion early. You can feel that your heart is racing and you can say to yourself, *Oh no, I'm becoming angry. I'm operating under the influence of anger, almost as if it's a powerful drug.* Anger can be very destructive, primarily because of the kinds of behaviors it motivates, and often we take out our anger on the people we love. Someone can do something that pushes your buttons and you get really upset. Before you know it, you have said something you wish you had not said. If you have been practicing, however, you can feel it happening and you can notice that you are operating under the influence of anger. You realize it is better not to say that thing, and you do not say it. You just let the energy of the anger run its course. It is not a matter of trying to push it away—just let it run its course. The energy can and will subside.

Thus, meditation can make a huge difference for emotions in several ways. One is this aspect of calming down, and the other is mindfulness, because it can play a role right from the very beginning in how you encounter events, in how you might typically respond to certain situations. Rather than having an automatic, quick appraisal, maybe you can slow that down and see that the situation is not threatening. Appraisal is one stage where mindfulness has a huge impact. One of the things that I do when I teach meditation, and it is the same in Mindfulness-Based Stress Reduction, is to encourage people to feel the emotion or stress in the body. If you can notice it and feel it, it can be incredibly informative. If you can see, for example, that you are starting to feel frightened, it tells you something about the sense you have made of the situation. Then you can ask yourself, *Why am I scared to walk in here? What is threatening here?* One of the things about meditation is this element of analyzing and inquiring in some sense into how you work, and in that process you are learning about yourself. So mindfulness is helpful at every stage of the emotion process, from appraisal through response.

I would also like to underline the importance of loving-kindness and compassion. When I talk about happiness with my students, I often define it as "being increasingly okay with whatever arises in life." That might sound rather boring and realistic, but when we talk about happiness we are not necessarily talking about the momentary joyousness or exultation that can occur in a certain situation. What we really mean is, *Are you well? Are things going okay? Can you move through life in a way that feels good?* In order to be happy, you have to be able to be gentle with yourself, to be okay with yourself, and to have a sense of humor about your own shortcomings. Then a lightness and humor develop. We have all met people who have this light, joyous quality about them. The more you are able to go easy on yourself, the happier you will be. These qualities can be cultivated as well.

Of course, most practices are based on cultivating compassion for others, and on being more gentle and non-harmful, and counteracting anger and destructive states. But tenderness and care for *oneself* are key in being able to let go of the sources of suffering in life. One of the big problems with all the misery and suffering that we experience around emotions is that we cannot let go of things; we grasp them ceaselessly. We perseverate, and we hold on to the source of aversion or upset. The cultivation of mindfulness and self-compassion allows us to calm down, to see that we are doing this, and to remember, *I want to be happy and have the sources of happiness. I want to be free from suffering and the sources of suffering.* If you have worked with this and you have really internalized it, then you say to yourself, *Right! I don't want to be miserable. What am I doing*? With practice, this can become an increasingly automatic reaction.

If I had to say in one or two sentences what the benefits of meditation were for your whole life—for your emotional life in particular—it is that meditative practice helps introduce the element of choice. Emotions seem unbidden, as though they happen to us and we are overcome and cannot do anything about them. But we can modify this—we can calm down, we can learn to see, we can learn to lighten up—and that is huge. We cannot necessarily control what the outside world offers us, but we can control how we respond to it. That is the element of choice, and choice creates freedom.

I have explained in some detail how my study of emotions has infused my thinking in meditation practice and teaching, but I will now discuss how practice has played a role in how I conduct myself as a scientist, and the way I ask questions. When we study emotions in the context of the Shamatha Project—and we are just beginning to understand the data there—one area that we are looking at is whether cultivating calm, clarity, and qualities of heart has an effect on the types of emotions that we have in response to different situations. But we are also extremely interested in whether it increases our awareness of emotions as they unfold. When you practice meditation regularly, you can begin to slow down the emotional process. You can see an emotion emerge and you know what you are feeling when it comes up, rather than later on when you reflect back on it. To my knowledge, nobody has really studied this in a laboratory.

One of the studies that we carried out as part of the Shamatha Project was to show people disturbing films and to measure their facial expressions and carry out very detailed ratings of their experience. One of the reasons for doing this was that we wanted to see if we could get a picture of people's emotions as they were going through them. The question was, Can we test whether meditation makes us more accurate observers of our own emotions? Any meditation practitioner will reply, "Of course it does!" But we thought it would be fascinating if we could get some scientific evidence for that, and so we set out to elicit emotions, and we measured experience and behavior over time.[2]

How can one evaluate whether we can become more accurate observers of our emotions? The only way that we know to find out what people think they are feeling is to ask them. Immediately after watching the film, participants in the study were asked to provide a fairly detailed emotional profile of what they felt throughout, so that we had an ongoing record. We did not want to ask while they were watching the film what they felt, because if you are reporting your feelings while you are watching something, it makes it hard to watch it in the first place. In addition, by breaking down and analyzing people's facial expressions as they changed over time, almost frame by frame, we had a dynamic measure of behavior, which served as an objective indicator of what they were going through. We expect that the meditators who did the intensive retreat will show greater coherence or agreement between what their faces were showing (an objective index of emotion) and what they said they were feeling throughout the film. In other words, we are expecting their reports of their emotions to be more accurate than those of the controls.

We do not have the findings on this congruence yet, but if our data support our hypothesis, it will give us the first scientific evidence that we can learn to see emotions as they happen. You need to do that if you are to have a choice as to how to respond, and that is the essence of the freedom or liberation of decoupling set emotional reactions from given situations in our lives. When people have that information, can they make choices about their emotions in time? It would be great to test this question empirically, but I have yet to think about how you would test this in a laboratory. That is something we would like to look at next.

I would like to end with a quotation from my teacher, Tarthang Tulku Rinpoche. In his book, *Openness Mind*, there is a wonderful section where he describes how we try to avoid emotions because we find them so frustrating. Instead, he says, we should welcome them. This is actually very common in the Tibetan tradition, to welcome emotions as opportunities for transformation and growth. "Emotions show us where to direct our attention. Rather than obscure the path, they can clarify and sharpen it."[3]

In other words, emotions tell us about what matters to us. They show us where we need to work, and if we can learn from that, we can reflect back and think more about the choices that we make and the opportunities that we have for greater happiness and freedom from suffering.

6

Meditation and Neuroscience

Sara Lazar, PhD

Have you ever wondered what goes on inside someone's head during meditation? The neuroscientist Sara Lazar uses an MRI scanner to measure brain activity and investigate how regular practice can alter the structure of a meditator's brain. She presents some of her most recent research, which has shown that meditation changes parts of the brain responsible for processing emotions, and has a powerful effect on the amygdala, the brain's trigger for fear, stress, and anger.

For more than two thousand years it has been claimed that meditation can bring about a wide range of positive effects, for both the body and the mind. Only much more recently, however, has the scientific community begun to unveil empirically the numerous beneficial changes that occur while one is meditating, including decreases in stress hormones and increases in biological markers of physical relaxation.

Beyond the more immediate effects of meditation, practitioners also report experiencing longer-lasting effects. Although it is said that the sense of calm and clarity that often persists throughout the day is not as intense as during formal sitting in meditation, practitioners frequently report that following meditation practice they are better able to navigate and cope with difficult situations or emotions, and that they have increased empathy and compassion, as well as improved memory and ability to pay attention. Several scientific groups have begun to test these claims, and good scientific evidence now exists to support some of them, particularly for attention and compassion. However, it is still not clear exactly how the practice of meditation leads to these widespread effects, and in particular, what neural mechanisms may underlie these beneficial changes. The goal of my research, therefore, is to understand how meditation practice may be impacting the brain, and how these brain changes may in turn lead to long-lasting benefits.

Here I broadly define behavior as actions of both the body and the mind. Under this umbrella, the aspects of human experience that meditators claim can be changed with practice, such as emotions, attention, or intention, can all be defined as behaviors. From a neuroscientific perspective all behavior is dependent on brain activity, which is dependent on brain structure. Brain structure can be very loosely defined as anything related to the way neurons communicate with each other, from the number of connections between neurons to the amount of neurotransmitter that is released between them. It is generally believed that to have a long-lasting shift in behavior, there must be a corresponding change in brain structure. For example, when you learn a new piece of information, changes occur in your brain structure as the information is encoded into memory. The following day those neurons will fire in a new way, which will allow you to recall the information. This process is known as neuroplasticity.

Another way to change brain structure is to repeat a behavior many times. Each time you do this, you trigger a cascade of corresponding brain activity, and over time these patterns become automatic and encoded differently than random behaviors. This is how habits form.

Neuroplasticity is at the heart of the therapeutic process as well as the learning process. If a depressed patient goes to see a doctor, the doctor might prescribe antidepressive medication, which will alter the patient's brain structure. Regular intake of the medication will change the amount of neurotransmitter being released into or removed from the space between neurons. That in turn affects the patient's brain activity, which brings about changes in behavior, namely a less depressive mood. If the same patient were to see a psychotherapist, he or she might engage in talk therapy. The therapist might challenge some of the patient's beliefs and self-doubts, or encourage the patient to look at situations from a different perspective. If these techniques are successful, some change in brain structure or function will accompany this change in perspective or attitude. The work of Helen Mayberg and colleagues gives some interesting examples of this.[1]

In my research, I set out to investigate what happens if you regularly engage in meditation for forty minutes a day for several years. If meditation can lead to long-lasting changes in mood, attention, and other behaviors, then it should be possible to observe changes in brain structure that are specific to meditation, and these changes should be related to shifts in behavior.

My tool of choice for examining the effects of meditation practice on brain structure and function is the magnetic resonance imaging (MRI) scanner. The scanner is a large tube encircled by powerful magnets that can detect small changes in magnetization inside the brain that naturally occur as a person's mind shifts between tasks. Two different types of images can be made with the MRI scanner: functional and structural. Functional MRI images capture changes in whichever part of the brain is active in real time. When someone is engaging in a particular task, we can observe on the scan which parts of the brain are active during that task, relative to the brain at rest or when performing other tasks. In contrast, structural MRI images reveal how much gray matter is present in different parts of the brain. By comparing images of a participant's brain structure captured prior to learning how to meditate and then again several weeks later, we are able to detect any changes that occurred as a result of meditation practice.

In 2005 we conducted a study with twenty practitioners of Theravada meditation. These were lay practitioners rather than monks or nuns, although to take part in the research they had to have completed at least one eight-day silent retreat and had to meditate for forty minutes each day, at least five days a week. We also had fifteen control subjects who were matched with the meditators for gender, age, education, and race, but had no experience of practicing meditation.

While the meditators were in the MRI scanner, we scanned their brains as they practiced "breath awareness meditation," and also while they were awake but not focusing their attention on any particular task. Our research showed that certain parts of the brain were clearly active during meditation. This was not the case when the subjects were simply resting and not doing anything in particular with their minds. One of the main criticisms that meditation researchers have received in the past is that we do not know whether the subject is actually meditating—maybe they are just relaxing or maybe even falling asleep. So it was important for us to be able to compare activity during meditation to activity during rest, to show clearly that these states are different.

The regions of the brain in which we found increased activity during meditation were the insula, the temporal pole, and the anterior cingulate cortex. These three regions together form the paralimbic cortex. To put it simply, the limbic system is the emotional center of your brain, whereas the cortical regions are engaged during thinking and problem solving. The paralimbic cortex connects these regions, and very loosely speaking can be thought of as the "mind-body connection" part of the brain. It is interesting that these regions have been implicated in numerous psychiatric diseases, including anxiety disorders, depression, bipolar disorder, and schizophrenia.

Another finding that we uncovered within the group of meditators was that there was decreased activity in a part of the brain called the amygdala, which is a core component of the neural network responsible for the so-called fight or flight response. Decreased activity is consistent with a decrease in arousal and an increase in the sense of well-being, which is a commonly reported effect of meditation.

Next, we investigated brain structure by measuring the amount of gray matter. Gray matter is the parts of the brain where neurons talk to each other and where "thinking" and neural activity actually happen; white matter is the parts of the brain made up of long-distance fibers that carry information from one part of the brain to another.

Our core question was, Does gray matter change as a result of meditation practice? We were led to this inquiry by several studies that compared specific groups of people and found group differences in gray matter. One study looked at bilingual individuals and found that those who learn a second language as a young child have significantly more gray matter in brain regions associated with language than those who learn a second language as a teenager, or individuals who only speak one language. Another study found that professional musicians have more gray matter than amateur musicians in areas of the brain related to musical ability, and that the amateurs had more gray matter than people with no musical training. In both of these studies, the amount of gray matter correlated with proficiency or experience.[2]

Another study investigated brain plasticity through the lens of juggling. The investigators recruited individuals who had never juggled before, scanned their brains, and then taught them how to juggle. The subjects were instructed to juggle every day for three months. After three months, they were scanned a second time, at which point they were told to stop juggling. Three months later, they were scanned for a third time. It was found that after three months of juggling, the region of the brain that is involved in detecting motion had increased in size. When they subsequently stopped juggling, the same region of the brain decreased in size. It was a classic example of "use it or lose it."[3]

The results of this research led us to hypothesize that if changes could occur in three months, then there should be differences in the brains of our subjects, who had all been practicing meditation for many years, when compared with a control group. When we performed the analyses we found that there were indeed parts of the gray matter that were thicker in the meditators than in the control group. The main region in which we found this difference was the insula, one of the paralimbic regions involved in the integration of senses, emotions, and thoughts. The insula in particular is involved in awareness of visceral processes, such as heart rate, breathing rate, and hunger. This region has also been found to be active in monks when they are engaging in compassion practices. Additionally, the insula has been found to be physically smaller in schizophrenic and bipolar patients than in healthy control subjects.[4]

We also found significantly more gray matter in part of the prefrontal cortex, which is involved in working memory and selective attention. It is well known that this part of the brain decreases in thickness as we age. Interestingly, when we plotted each person's cortical thickness in this region against their age, the graph suggested that meditation may help to slow down or even prevent this normal age-related decline in thickness. Our cortex is at its thickest in our early to mid-twenties, then gradually thins as we get older. In this one very small area of the brain, however, the forty- and fifty-year-old meditators had the same level of cortical thickness as the twenty-year-old subjects. Our findings suggest that the forty- to fifty-year-old subjects may have prevented decay in this region of their brains by frequently activating it through meditation practice. This research leads to some potentially exciting lines of inquiry, although it still needs to be replicated.

Critics were not satisfied with these results, and we received comments and feedback along the lines of, "Meditators are 'different'; their brains were probably like that before they even started." Or, "Maybe it's because they rested for forty minutes every day, or because they are vegetarian, or something else about their lifestyle that is different to that of the controls." These are valid points, and our data set was not able to address them directly. Still, there are a few things to note. The first point is that the insula was the main area of the brain we found to be active during meditation. If an individual is activating the insula for forty minutes each day through meditation practice, it is logical to expect this to lead to increases in the amount of gray matter in this region of the brain. A second important point is that the pattern we observed was highly localized. Studies have shown that factors such as diet exhibit effects across the entire brain that are not highly localized. In contrast, our results were consistent with the idea that meditation has a very specific effect on the parts of the brain that are engaged during meditation practice.

Four other groups have since conducted experiments similar to ours, using long-term meditators and control groups. However, each study used subjects who practiced in different lineages of Buddhist meditation, and each study had different criteria for how much the subjects needed to have practiced meditation, or the age of the subjects who were included. All of these factors can influence results. Also, the studies did not use identical methods for analyzing gray matter, and it is known that the measurement method used can identify different regions of gray matter differences. Consequently, it is difficult to compare directly the results of the studies' findings. However, two of the studies have found a difference between the size of the hippocampus of the meditation practitioners and of the control subjects.[5] The method I used in my study was optimized to detect differences specifically in the cortex, and did not enable us to look at subcortical structures such as the hippocampus.

The hippocampus is primarily involved in emotion regulation, learning, and memory. It is a particularly interesting region, as it is sensitive to cortisol, a steroid hormone that is released in response to stress. Prolonged exposure to elevated levels of cortisol can have detrimental effects on the neuronal cells in your brain. The hippocampus also generates new neurons throughout a person's entire life, and excessive cortisol levels prevent the neurons from being regenerated. Our neuroimaging findings with meditators and controls suggest that meditation practice may hold the potential to prevent the detrimental effects of stress on the brain, which has important implications for numerous psychological conditions where the structure and function of the hippocampus are important, such as depression and post-traumatic stress disorder.

Studying people who have practiced meditation for many years can provide valuable insights into how meditation works. However, it is important to verify these findings by testing whether similar types of changes occur when novices learn how to meditate. In our second study we recruited individuals from Jon Kabat-Zinn's mindfulness clinic in Worcester, Massachusetts, who were about to undergo the eight-week Mindfulness-Based Stress Reduction (MBSR) program.[6] This highly structured program focuses on training participants in core mindfulness and meditative practices. We conducted MRI scans both before participants entered the course and after they completed it. We compared the imaging data collected from the participants with a group of people who were on a wait-list to take the program a few months later. We found gray matter increases in the hippocampus, a region called the posterior cingulate cortex, and a region called the temporal-parietal junction. Gray matter in the insula also increased, though the difference was not statistically significant. As I mentioned, the hippocampus is integral to learning and memory, the posterior cingulate cortex is involved with self-processing—how what you encounter day to day relates to you—and the temporal-parietal junction plays a central role in empathy and compassion.

In the mindfulness group, we also found that there was a decrease in the gray matter density of the amygdala, which, interesting to note, was correlated with a change in perceived stress levels.

The greater the decrease in a participant's stress levels, the less dense the amygdala was following the mindfulness intervention. The amygdala is integral to the fight or flight response, so this change is consistent with the known biology.[7]

Our findings in the amygdala have important parallels with studies conducted on rats in which it was found that after the animals were placed in a stressful living situation, the amygdala of the rats had become more dense. The researchers then put the rats back in a nonstressful environment. When they tested the rats again three weeks later, the amygdala remained more dense and the animals behaved as though they were under stress. Their environment changed, but not their brains or their behavior.[8] This was the opposite situation for our subjects. Following the eight-week mindfulness intervention, their lives were still the same; they still had the same stressful jobs and the same difficult people in their lives. Their environment had not changed, but their brains and their relationship to their environment had. The decreased size of the amygdala is a reflection of this internal shift. It is notable that this observed neural plasticity may be a reflection of a shift in attitude and perspective, and not rooted in environmental factors.

Unfortunately, we do not know exactly what causes these changes in gray matter. We do know that neurons are formed in the hippocampus, so changes in this region may be due to this. But the mechanism of change for the other regions of the brain is uncertain. It may be due to an increase or decrease in the number of connections between the neurons in the affected regions. Alternatively, gray matter is supported by small helper cells called astrocytes, as well as by blood vessels. In animal studies it has been shown that changes in gray matter resulting from learning are often associated with increases in the number of helper cells or the size of blood vessels. A change in any of these three is consistent with physiological underpinnings of acquiring new information. As we cannot distinguish between these three types of neural changes using MRI technology, it is unclear whether the changes that we observed in the brain were due to new connections or to helper cells or blood vessels. We just know that changes in gray matter take place.

To summarize, our research on meditators has revealed structural changes in regions of the brain that are important for emotion regulation, empathy, and self-referential processing. Furthermore, changes in stress levels correlated with changes in amygdala gray matter density. These data provide important information on how meditation works, and lend considerable evidence to the claims of meditators that practice improves their mood, their emotion regulation capacity, and, in particular, their ability to handle stressful situations. This is just the tip of the iceberg though, as there is still much to learn about how these brain changes lead to the myriad changes that meditators report.

I am frequently asked, "Are these data telling us that people should meditate to make their brains bigger?" Or, "I'm getting older, should I meditate to stop my brain from shrinking?" Although our data show that the brain does change with meditation practice, it is important to remember that learning any new task will lead to changes in your brain. The point of the data is to start to learn how meditation may be working. However, I have heard from many meditation teachers that when people first come to classes, they are often a little skeptical. Students ask, "Is this really doing anything for me?" Or, "Do I need to practice for many years to get the positive benefits of meditation?" One use of the data is to help diminish these doubts concerning the efficacy of meditation and mindfulness, as opposed to presenting the brain changes as an incentive.

I will leave you with a Zen koan: "Intending to buy iron, they obtain gold." In my own case, I started practicing yoga as a form of physical therapy for knee pain. I didn't believe any of the health or cognitive claims that the teacher made, but after a few weeks I realized that there was much more to yoga practice than just a way to rehabilitate my knee. This is a common experience for those coming to meditation and meditation practices. They begin practice looking for stress reduction, or to increase their brain size, or to bring some other tangible benefit to their life. But they start to realize that these practices do much more, that they enrich their lives in inexplicable ways and help them in ways that they didn't even know they needed to be helped.

PART THREE

Mindfulness in Health Care

7

Mindfulness-Based Interventions in Medicine and Psychiatry

What Does It Mean to Be "Mindfulness-Based"?

Jon Kabat-Zinn, PhD

A scientist, author, and meditation teacher, Jon Kabat-Zinn is the man who put mindfulness on the map. The Mindfulness-Based Stress Reduction (MBSR) program that he developed has spread from its initial home in a hospital basement in Worcester, Massachusetts, to medical institutions around the world. Who better than the program's founder to explain how mindfulness came into mainstream health care, share its rationale and key principles, and outline how he expects the confluence of medicine and meditation to evolve in the future?

It is a very radical step—I would even say a revolutionary one—to organize a forum on meditation and health and to bring the worlds of medicine and neuroscience into a Tibetan Buddhist temple. We are on very delicate ground here. We are stretching the limits of our understanding and discourse in bringing together two extraordinary worlds that, for the first time in history, are speaking to each other and inquiring together in thoughtful and open ways about areas of overlapping interest, as well as perhaps illuminating significant and important differences in certain viewpoints and approaches. This is how further learning and understanding come about in the human community.

This confluence of science and both "big D" and "little d" Dharma has never before happened in history.* It offers a profound opportunity for exploring different epistemologies, in other words, different ways of knowing and different methodologies for systematically investigating, through both observation and experiment, outwardly and through introspection, the nature of reality and its potential to reduce human suffering.[1] The mutual engagement of these different ways of knowing has the potential to transform our understanding of health and well-being, of disease and dis-ease, of the nature of the mind and its relationship to the body and the domain of the heart. These are all deep inquiries that no single discipline has the last word or the inside track on. So perhaps there is some potential for our explorations to give rise to what I like to call an "orthogonal rotation in consciousness"—a new way of perceiving reality by shifting reference frames by 90 degrees, much like when we put two polarized filters on top of each other, see that the light is blocked, and then rotate one 90 degrees with respect to the other and light comes through. In an orthogonal relationship, different perspectives can interpenetrate and give rise, if held in awareness, to a rotation in consciousness. In that moment of seeing, everything is different and new degrees of freedom and possibility open up, offering new dimensions—and yet everything is also the exactly the same.[2]

---

* By "big D" Dharma, I mean the Buddhadharma. By "little d" dharma, I mean the same teachings in essence but in a universal language and forms that are not framed as Buddhist but simply as human.

For many people, such as those we see as medical patients in the stress-reduction clinic at the University of Massachusetts Medical Center, it probably would not be appropriate or wise to invite them into a space like Lerab Ling—a magnificent Tibetan Buddhist temple, with its gigantic and imposing golden Buddha—and then attempt to introduce them to the work that my colleagues and I are engaged in, the meditative cultivation of mindfulness, even though mindfulness is often spoken of as *the heart of Buddhist meditation.* It might not come across as of universal applicability or particularly relevant to them, were they to encounter it in this form.

Mindfulness-Based Stress Reduction, or MBSR, is designed to teach people with medical problems and more generally with stress, pain, and illness how to take better care of themselves and move toward greater levels of health and well-being through the cultivation and systematic practice of mindfulness meditation. From my perspective, and from my understanding of the Dharma, it is neither necessary nor wise to expose people in such an explicit and dramatic way to the Buddhist roots of mindfulness. In some sense, there is something already present in all of us that does not need any of the cultural forms that surround us in a space like Lerab Ling. The forms are beautiful, and I love them myself, but they could be impediments to understanding the relevance and benefits of what we might call "little *d*" dharma for the majority of people on the planet who are suffering and who could benefit from training in mindfulness in a more universal idiom and form. That is precisely what MBSR is meant to be. Most people would probably see the iconography and architecture here as representing a religion, which, of course, they do. People justifiably might say, "Why should I engage in Buddhist practices, or adopt a belief system foreign to my culture?" But if all this is framed universally, even though the connection to Buddhist meditation practices is made quite explicit when appropriate, it can present a significantly lower barrier for engaging. After all, paying attention is hardly Buddhist. Nor are awareness, kindness, compassion, or wisdom. My understanding and experience of the Dharma remind me that the essence of the dharma and how it is practiced are absolutely formless. If that is so, then we can ask what the most skillful means might be for cultivating liberative insight and embodiment in ways that obviate any and all barriers to cultivating, and ultimately embodying, wisdom, compassion, and kindness.

Sogyal Rinpoche points to the value and power of nonattachment, of clear seeing, of resting in the original nature of mind, in the boundless spaciousness of awareness (see chapter 1). This perspective seems to be already universal in essence. It is also true that one could sit in any room—for example, in a conference room in our hospital—without any of the iconography that surrounds us in a temple and still not understand this essential point. It wouldn't make much sense and might sound like gobbledygook. You might be familiar with all the words being used—*awareness*, *compassion*, *sitting*—and yet still not understand what is being pointed to. To understand in a deep way, we have to be *moved*, we have to have an authentic *encounter*, we have to have a *taste* of a larger perspective on ourselves and our relationship to experience—and these only come by engaging in meditation practice in a regular and disciplined way. When we involve ourselves in daily practice, the words can begin to make some sense, because we are familiarizing ourselves with the nature of our own mind and our own experience. It becomes a firsthand or, to use Francisco Varela's term, a first-person experience.[3] Then we might be more open to receiving what is being offered through skillful teaching—because we are slowly, through the cultivation of mindfulness (which includes heartfulness), expanding our relationship with our own experience and looking more deeply into it. This can lead in different ways to that rotation in consciousness I mention above. Without a practice, we are much more likely to be caught up in our ideas and opinions without even knowing it. This is important, because our attachment to those ideas and opinions can prevent us from being in touch with the actuality of things. When you realize that a thought is just a thought and not the truth, there is a huge shift in how you understand your own mind. It is already a profound rotation in consciousness.

Everyone has the potential to explore this kind of creative interface within a universally articulated dharma. There is no catechism or dogma one needs to adhere to. If we understand that the exploration of one's own experience is entirely empirical, then the arc of developing one's own meditation practice and integrating it into one's life will be minimally freighted with cultural baggage and, therefore, relatively straightforward. The value in terms of its potential for transformation and liberation for ourselves and for others can at least be entertained as a plausible hypothesis, worthy of testing in one's own life through practice. Moreover, this kind of inclusive approach might have the potential to move out into the world in ways that could contribute to healing a great deal of the suffering writ large that we human beings bring upon ourselves and inflict upon one another at both a societal and a global level. Still, everybody needs to find his or her own way to engage in this adventure. There is no one size fits all, no single way to approach and inhabit awareness.

Biological science has made it completely clear by now, if there was any doubt, that there is no essential separation between what we call "mind" and what we call "body." With apologies to René Descartes, given that this conference is taking place in his home country, that kind of dualism is now defunct.[4]

We could say that mindfulness involves, as the Buddha said, being "a light unto yourself." You do not even have to *become* a light unto yourself, because your very nature is already luminous. Images and statues of the Buddha do not represent a deity, strictly speaking, but rather a human being, one who was deeply committed to understanding the nature of his own suffering and of his own mind. It is said that people used to ask the Buddha, "Are you a god?" His response was, "No, I am awake." That is one hell of a message. He is not differentiating himself from anybody else. Rather, he is pointing to the true nature of all of us—wakefulness itself or, more ordinarily, awareness, when it is fully embodied. You do not have to be Buddhist to embody wakefulness or to cultivate mindfulness. It is more a matter of recognizing your essential buddha nature right now—that you are already a buddha. And because in essence that is already what you are, there is nothing to resist or to attain. There is no problem. The only challenge is whether you can live this actuality in any single moment, whether you can embody this recognition and allow it to suffuse and saturate your entire being. Mindfulness is not about *trying* to make anything happen. It is about recognizing and allowing that dimensionality of your being, that quality of wakefulness with no agenda or self-involvement, to be at the forefront of your relationship with life rather than totally hidden away, unnoticed and unused.

When I started the pilot program for what rapidly became the stress-reduction clinic at the University of Massachusetts Medical Center in 1979, few people in the mainstream knew or used the word *mindfulness* to refer to a form of meditation practice, and even fewer knew or used the word *dharma.* There was virtually no interest in such things in medical and scientific circles. For some time, I had been asking myself how I could bring my own dharma practice together with right livelihood so that my work and training in science and my meditation practice might meld into one seamless whole and allow me to lead a more integrated life, and perhaps engage in something of intrinsic value to the world—something that has been here all along but is difficult at times for us to recognize or decode. I was not going to become a monastic—I had a wife and child and the strong intention to have a rich family life. How could I reconcile these two different dimensions of my life in such a way that my work and my dharma practice would be the same thing? I did not want to engage in some other kind of work to make a living, and then try to integrate my meditation practice into that life. I wanted the work itself to be grounded in, and about, meditation and its potential value. This was in part because I felt the world was starving for a more mindful way of being, and yet there was no obvious conventional way to be "gainfully employed" in such an undertaking; and it was in part because whatever our work and whatever our circumstances, the real meditation is life itself and how we choose to live it. It is not just sitting in a certain posture for a time, either using a particular object to focus on or in objectless attending. We really only get one moment to show up in our life—this one. Yet we rarely notice it because it is so easy to get distracted and drift out of touch. But if we are not inhabiting this present moment, then we are invariably lost in the past or obsessing about the future. We can drive ourselves crazy with fear and anxiety, and meanwhile the beauty of the present moment, the potential of this moment, and the potential for coming to terms with things as they are *in* this moment—which is actually my working definition of *healing*—are obliterated.

When we think about hospitals and their role in society, we might say that they function as *dukkha* magnets, drawing in people who are suffering, who are dealing with stress, pain of all kinds, disease, and illness.[5] Nobody goes to the hospital to have a good time. We usually go to the hospital when the pain and suffering become too intense to ignore or to tolerate without help. Hospitals are not the only dukkha magnets in society—schools, prisons, and the military could also be described this way. For that reason, there might be a profound role for mindfulness in transforming these institutions. There are now growing efforts to bring mindfulness into K–12 education, into the military, and into prisons, and to study the effects that such programs are having on the participants. Early indicators suggest that the outcomes of such trainings in these very different domains of life can be surprisingly profound and very much in the direction of greater harmony, peace, and learning, whether in the classroom, in war zones, or in the prison yard.

Some Buddhist scholars translate the word *dukkha* as "stress." When I used the label "stress reduction" to describe the training in mindfulness we were offering to our medical patients, embedded within it was the sense that we were addressing the entire scope of the human condition. The Buddhist framework of dukkha, the first Noble Truth, fits this context perfectly. So here is one interface between dharma and medicine, pointing to an understanding of the root causes of suffering. In fact, the Four Noble Truths were offered by the Buddha—who was often referred to as "the physician of the world"—in the form of a classical medical framework. The first

Noble Truth, that of dukkha—usually translated as suffering, anguish, unsatisfactoriness, dis-ease, or stress—is the *diagnosis*. The second Noble Truth is the *etiology* or ultimate cause of the dis-ease, namely clinging or self-identification. The third Noble Truth is the *prognosis*, in this case the possibility of a very good outcome indeed, namely freedom from suffering. And the fourth Noble Truth is in the form of a precise *treatment plan*, namely the Eightfold Noble Path, of which mindfulness is one of eight interacting and interpenetrating factors, and in MBSR is meant as a placeholder for all of them.[6]

Here is another conjunction between dharma and medicine. When you listen carefully, the words *meditation* and *medicine* sound a lot alike. Etymologically, they share a deep root meaning; meditation and medicine are joined at the hip, so to speak. Both are concerned with the same thing in the most profound way—liberation from suffering. The root of both words carries the meaning of *measure*, in the Platonic sense of everything having its own "right inward measure." Medicine is the restoring of right inward measure when it is disturbed, and meditation is the direct perception of right inward measure.[7] Meditation is something that we can practice inwardly and that can influence our relationship with experience, with the human condition itself. And it can also influence our relationship with our own stress, pain, and illness, especially when we run into the very real limits of modern medicine as we seek it out to help restore us to optimal health. Medicine allows us to benefit from external care when we need it, but of course in the long run the best medicine, when we can manage it, is preventive medicine.

Mindfulness-Based Stress Reduction was designed to function as a safety net to catch people falling through the cracks of the health-care system. It challenges them to do something for themselves that no one else—including their doctors, surgeons, pastors, and family members—could do for them, via the systematic cultivation of mindfulness through their own disciplined efforts, with huge encouragement and support from the clinic staff and their MBSR instructor.

In the United States, we tend to see ourselves as go-getters, as doers. So when your doctor refers you to a program where you are told that you will learn to be in relationship to your own experience—including, at times, extremely unpleasant and even painful experiences—and what is more, you will do this mostly in silence for extended periods of time, this invitation doesn't necessarily go over so well. Unless, that is, you really can meet the person exactly where he or she is and connect with his or her pain and aspirations in a deep way. The business world would call this kind of invitation a "hard sell." But what if people are actually starving for stillness, for learning how to inhabit *the domain of being*?[8] What if learning how to inhabit silence and stillness and awareness—especially when you do so with kindness, with patience, and with self-compassion—is itself healing? Why not try to study this kind of question systematically and scientifically?

In our everyday lives, we tend to be so strongly committed to getting things done, to checking things off our endless to-do lists, to doing, doing, and more doing, that maybe we should call ourselves "human doings" rather than "human beings." Perhaps it is fair to say that we have forgotten how to be, except maybe on vacation for a few weeks a year. Very strange, don't you think? If you look around the animal kingdom, all the other creatures seem to know how to be. Frogs know how to be frogs, and insects know how to be insects. You never see a bird in flight suddenly become confused, get its wings tangled up, and fall out of the air. But we see ourselves and others getting caught up and lost in thought all the time. It is almost our default mode. If we are not careful, we might even walk into a door we are in the process of opening. We may be in such a hurry to get through it but so lost in thought that we don't realize we haven't completely opened it yet. I have certainly had that experience. It is an example of running on autopilot, of not being fully present and embodied in the only moment we are ever alive in, namely this one. MBSR is a systematic training program for inhabiting the present moment more reliably and for reclaiming the full dimensionality of our lives in the face of "the full catastrophe" of the human condition, a phrase spoken by the title character in the movie of Nikos Kazantzakis's novel *Zorba the Greek*. MBSR offers training in the cultivation of mindfulness for people facing stress, pain, and illness in their lives, which is all of us, sooner or later.

When I use the word *mindfulness*, I do not mean it in the usual way Buddhist teachers in some traditions use it. For instance, I do not mean it simply as the mental factor that knows whether the mind is on or off a particular object of attention. I intentionally use it in a number of different ways. I realized back in 1979 that if I were to get into differentiating between all the various perspectives on the meaning of mindfulness and its cultivation in different traditions, whether it is the perspective articulated in the Abhidharma[9] or the non-dual Mahayana understanding,[10] nobody would have been interested, and indeed most people would in all likelihood have become both confused and discouraged from practicing formal meditation. But while most people are simply not interested in such distinctions, they are very much interested in suffering and the possibility of liberation from suffering—especially, but not exclusively, their own.

So when I use the word *mindfulness*, in addition to using it as a synonym for *awareness*, I am using it as an umbrella term to include the entirety of the dharma in its most universal and non-dual essence, but not expressed as Buddhadharma. His Holiness the Dalai Lama talks about Buddhadharma and universal dharma as manifestations of common human values.[11] My strategy from the beginning was that once we reached the point where mindfulness had penetrated the mainstream of society to a significant degree, then perhaps the climate would be receptive for scholars to debate the subject and help us clarify and understand issues related to it in increasingly subtle ways. That time is now here, so I hope that these conversations will continue, as evidenced by the collection of papers in Williams and Kabat-Zinn (see note 1), first published as a Special Issue on Mindfulness in the journal *Contemporary Buddhism*. In particular, there are two papers by John Teasdale and

Michael Chaskalson that specifically address this interface of science and dharma, and the psychological and biological mechanisms by which the cultivation of mindfulness might be exerting its effects.[12]

To be explicit, to a first approximation, *mindfulness* as I use the term includes the full dimensionality of the dharma. At least it is meant to be that, and to signify pure awareness—the foundational nature of mind, the essence of mind. In Buddhist terms, it includes all four of the *Brahmaviharas*, the "four immeasurables" or virtues—loving-kindness, compassion, empathetic joy, and equanimity—as well as *shamatha* and *vipassana*.

Sometimes I say to people who do not know anything about Buddhism that MBSR teaches Buddhist meditation without the Buddhism. If you know anything about Buddhism, you realize that ultimately all Buddhist meditation is without the Buddhism. It is really about being human and realizing the full nature of our humanity, rather than identifying with a particular tradition, belief system, or set of customs, however wonderful they might be. If the mind, in some absolute way, makes "Buddhists" and "non-Buddhists," then it has created a certain kind of dualism and separation. And since the dharma is in essence non-dual, you are already in trouble! And let's not forget, the Buddha himself was not a Buddhist.

There is no intention whatsoever to be irreverent in saying this. I have great respect for the traditions and the wisdom they represent and have kept alive for millennia. I have practiced and grown up in the traditions. I have been nested and nurtured within them, and continue to be, and I very much honor my many teachers, more than I can express. At the same time, I feel there is something fascinating going on with Buddhism nowadays. On the one hand, in the West classical temples such as Lerab Ling are being built in the traditional way. On the other hand, as with the Buddhism and Medicine conferences it is sponsoring and hosting, it is clear that at least this temple is also serving as a container for a transformative interaction between worlds, the confluence of epistemologies I have been speaking about. Clearly this conference is designed to reach people who would never ordinarily walk into a place like Lerab Ling. The potential for transformation, for all of us to learn and to grow, is therefore enormous. At the same time, there is also the potential for colossal misunderstandings if we are not clear about how we pursue such opportunities going forward, after a conference such as this one. So it is stretching everybody, all of us, not just the non-Buddhists.

I once had an extended talk with a Chinese Chan master, Venerable Bun Huan, in Shenzhen. He was ninety-eight years old at the time of my visit. He died recently at the age of 106. His Dharma heir explained to him what I did, after which he said to me, and the others gathered in the room, "There are an infinite number of ways in which people suffer. Therefore, there have to be an infinite number of ways in which the Dharma is made available."[13]

His Holiness the Dalai Lama said much the same thing when he first heard about MBSR during a Mind and Life Dialogue meeting in Dharamsala, India, in 1990.[14] Someone had raised, in a rather ominous way, the question of whether MBSR might be the beginning of the death knell of Buddhism. The implication was that the work we were doing was single-handedly going to, in some small but not insignificant way, pull the rug out from under 2,500 years of Buddhism by "secularizing" and "cherry-picking" favorite elements of a sacred whole, and ignoring other important aspects—including, it was suggested, the ethical and moral foundations of the religion. I knew from informal conversations among the presenters that the subject would be raised the next day, following my presentation. I sat up all night in what was formerly His Holiness's mother's house, Kashmir Cottage, where a number of us were staying, wondering what I would do if the Dalai Lama said I should shut down our clinic because it was going to contribute to undermining Buddhism. By morning, it was clear to me that although I have enormous respect for His Holiness, were he to say that MBSR was dangerous or harmful to Buddhism, I would still have to give priority to what our patients were saying and demonstrating about its value to them, as well as to my own experience. In the end, however, when asked about the dangers to the religion of introducing elements of its meditative practices and perspectives into the mainstream of medicine and the broader society, His Holiness responded, "There are four billion people on the planet. One billion are Buddhist; all four billion are suffering." That was all he said.[15]

The implication was clear. If there is any value to the dharma, it cannot be kept exclusively for Buddhists. All of us are suffering and need to understand suffering and its causes, and the potential for liberation from suffering through understanding the mind. So what else could one do except to try to find imaginative, creative, and authentic ways of bringing this way of being, this way of embodied awareness, of wisdom and kindness, to the people who need it the most and do not even know that they need it—and who would certainly not pursue it in a Buddhist temple like this one? What we are doing in some sense might be thought of as a recontextualization of dharma. However, it is not at all a decontextualization of the dharma, nor an abandoning of its fundamental ethical roots.

People everywhere are suffering from stress, pain, chronic illness—dukkha of every kind—and the suffering seems to begin at younger and younger ages. When I was a boy, in the 1950s, the onset of major clinical depression usually came in a person's fifties or sixties. Now it is happening at fourteen or fifteen years of age or even younger. Studies of the age of onset of major depression over time show that it has been occurring at progressively younger ages since the early part of the twentieth century. Indeed, depression is now a problem of epidemic proportions, and nobody really understands its causes. Here is another poignant measure of it: At the same Mind and Life Dialogue that I described above, Sharon Salzberg, a well-known and highly respected American vipassana teacher and author, matter-of-factly used the term *low self-esteem* while presenting to the Dalai Lama. All the Westerners in the room understood it, but none of the Tibetans had the faintest idea what we were talking about. It took about an hour to explain to His Holiness that in the West, many people do not feel good about themselves. It was an amazing cross-cultural revelation.[16]

MBSR was designed to serve as a dharma vehicle that includes the arc of ongoing self-development,* understanding, and wisdom. Mindfulness is not a Band-Aid. It is not a relaxation technique. It is not a technique at all. It is a way of being. There are hundreds of methods, hundreds of skillful means for cultivating greater awareness. The methods themselves are not important. What is important is the understanding of the potential for deep seeing into the nature of suffering and the nature of mind, and then for liberation from that suffering. Many of our patients come to understand this out of their own direct experiences with the formal meditation practices and their applications in everyday living. We do not have to spell it out for them. They may come to class after a week of practice and report, "Wow, I embraced my pain for the first time and it changed!" Sometimes they say it went away entirely, at least for a time. An experience like that can shift your relationship to the possible, and to how you are in relationship to your own body and mind, and to suffering in all the various ways that it manifests in the body, the mind, and the heart. Suddenly you see and understand more and, as a consequence, may actually take your own experience less personally. Your relationship to the interior narrative about your own experience and its meaning can change profoundly. It may gradually become a bit less self-centered and self-preoccupied. That in itself can be quite freeing, even if nothing else changes. It is transformative.

In fact, it is not uncommon for participants in MBSR and other mindfulness-based interventions to report changes in a number of domains in their lives that go far beyond their original hopes and expectations for participating in a mindfulness-based clinical program. This phenomenon is underscored by the subtitle of one recent paper on MBCT (Mindfulness-Based Cognitive Therapy): "It Changed Me in Just about Every Way Possible."[17] Put otherwise, people sometimes say things like, "This program gave me back my life."

---

* The term *bhavana* in Pali, often translated as "meditation," literally means "development" or "cultivation."

There is a paradox here, because when people come to the stress-reduction clinic, referred by their physicians or by family or friends for specific medical diagnoses and ailments, they are certainly not coming for enlightenment or to transform their entire life. The term *enlightenment* is not a part of their vocabulary or a motive for enrolling in MBSR. They come because they are hurting. They want to have their pain go away, or at least to learn how to live with it. They want to have their blood pressure drop or their T-cell count go up, or to have greater peace of mind. There are all sorts of reasons behind their motivations for coming. We say to them that the best way to promote the kind of changes they do hope for—or improvements of any kind for that matter—is, paradoxically, not to try to get anywhere at all but simply follow the meditation instructions with both resolve and a light and gentle touch, and just see what happens. Often transformation happens across a much wider range of domains than the person was expecting or even felt was possible. Sometimes it is a larger understanding of who one is—beyond the stories, the personal narratives, the attachment to the personal pronouns. It is important that this domain not be excluded from the range of possible outcomes. Indeed, it is an essential element of MBSR.

When it comes to mindfulness itself, there are many different views of what it is and what it is not. Even serious Buddhist scholars have disagreements, and have for centuries.[18] I have offered an operational definition of *mindfulness*: the awareness that arises by paying attention on purpose, in the present moment, and nonjudgmentally. It is not the last word on this subject, but it does point to how we can use our agency instrumentally to go from being on automatic pilot, or relatively mindless, to greater mindfulness. At the same time, it also points, through the verb *arises*, to the non-instrumental dimension, to the domain of non-doing, of being—which is at least as important as the instrumental dimension in recognizing and realizing our own wholeness.[19] Perhaps we could say that awareness itself is the final common pathway of our humanness and our humanity.

Paying attention in this way and learning to inhabit the awareness that arises from paying attention does not imply that you are a Buddhist. It simply reminds you of your humanity and allows you to embody it from moment to moment as a practice, if you can remember, which is itself another meaning of the term *mindfulness*, *sati* in Pali, the original language in which the teachings of the Buddha were written down.

The nonjudgmental aspect of our operational definition of mindfulness is key. It means having no aversion, or being aware of how aversive you may be in a particular moment. In Buddhist terms, we are talking about the second foundation of mindfulness, *vedena*, of being aware in the moment of contact with an arising of any kind, of whether it has the feeling tone of pleasant, unpleasant, or neither pleasant nor unpleasant. But we do not have to appeal formally to the four foundations of mindfulness, or even mention them in MBSR. We just pay attention, on purpose, in the present moment, nonjudgmentally. When I watch what is occurring in my own mind, judging of one kind or another is going on a great deal of the time. Being nonjudgmental does not mean that you should not have any judgments. It would be quite misleading to give people the impression that they had to be without any judgments. We all have ideas and opinions about everything, including ourselves, so it is not about *not having them*, it is about *embracing them in awareness* and therefore being in a different and more wise and flexible relationship with them.

We sometimes use the phrase "put out the welcome mat" to suggest how we might relate differently to our judging, or whatever else arises in our experience. For example, if you are meditating, and all of a sudden a strong feeling of some kind arises, let's say envy, you might feel bad about that or be critical of yourself. *I'm supposed to be meditating, but actually I'm driving myself crazy! I'm envious of somebody else's experience, and I shouldn't be.* But what if this experience were seen just as an arising, like a cloud? What if when such a feeling comes up you do not take it personally? You do not turn it into *I*, *me*, and *mine*. It is just another rising. We could watch it come and go. We could feel its effects in the body, and where they are most predominant. What if we could allow whatever arises in the present moment simply to be embraced in awareness—to just put out the welcome mat for it all?

Awareness is not disturbed by envy, jealousy, hatred, anger, depression, or more pleasant mind states either. It is characterized by equanimity. We are not promoting some kind of romantic idealism here. We are talking about whether in one moment it is possible simply to recognize the attachment to the concept of *I*, in relation to a feeling of envy. Then, for that moment at least, it would be a moment of liberation. As is sometimes said in the Dzogchen teachings on the essential nature of the mind and how to recognize it, thoughts liberate themselves. A simile I sometimes use when teaching what we call "choiceless awareness," or open presence, is that the self-liberation of thoughts is similar to when a soap bubble pops all by itself, or is touched by a finger. When thoughts or emotions arise—jealousy, anger, whatever it may be—the field of the mind, the field of awareness itself, has the effect of a finger touching a soap bubble. The thoughts self-liberate in awareness—except there is no finger and nobody to touch the bubble of thought, only awareness itself.

We give people plenty of space to learn about their relationship to their thoughts and emotions in MBSR, MBCT, and all the other mindfulness-based interventions that are developing now in education, in childbirth and parenting, in relapse prevention for alcohol addiction, in the military, in prisons, and so on. There are mindfulness-based interventions spreading around the world and they all have to do with embodying the full dimensionality of this practice. I am putting this whole development under the umbrella of "mindfulness," but it could be expressed in many different ways. The main point is that people have the opportunity to experience the healing power of their own attention and awareness, as both mindfulness and heartfulness, especially when these capacities are cultivated and refined through ongoing practice—and without the practitioners necessarily needing to know much, if anything, about the particular cultural origins of these practices or their philosophical underpinnings. The instructors, of course, do have to know and study this to some degree.

The dharma, whether with a little *d* or a big *D*, has a deep structure to it that needs to be the foundation out of which the instruction of mindfulness-based interventions comes. If we are calling something "mindfulness-based," then it really has to be mindfulness-based. And that means dharma-based. Mindfulness is not another cognitive-behavioral technique coming out of the Western psychological tradition. It is orthogonal to (at right angles and interpenetrating with) that tradition, and thus has huge potential to add to our basic understanding of ourselves as human beings, and to our understanding of the brain, the mind-body connection, and what we call "the self."

It is also important to emphasize that an ethical foundation undergirds the entire dharma, a clearly articulated understanding of what is harmful, and the conscious decision—even in the face of one's own mind's destructive emotions and impulses—not to harm. That is the ethical foundation of medicine as well: a core principle of the Hippocratic Oath is "First, do no harm." This is very much akin to the aspiration and commitment behind the Bodhisattva Vow. You surrender your own ambition, even your ambition to attain liberation or enlightenment, and you serve the greater good of all beings and their liberation from suffering in whatever ways are possible. You do this not in pursuit of an ideal but as an embodiment of your own truest nature as not separate, as interconnected with all beings, and thus impelled to act to relieve suffering. This is the basis of empathy and true compassion.

It is said that in most Asian languages, the words for *mind* and *heart* are the same. For this reason, I like to emphasize with English-speaking audiences—as I have already alluded to in several places—that when we hear the word *mindfulness*, if we are not simultaneously inwardly hearing *heartfulness*, then we are not really understanding what the word *mindfulness* is pointing to. When we hear *mind* we can easily get cerebral, conceptual, and perhaps a bit clinical, saying, "Oh, mindfulness, that's about such and such, like being present in the moment." Yes, that is true. But at the same time, there is much more to it. Mindfulness is fundamentally about freedom, about liberation—it is fully embodied awareness, or as Bhikkhu Bodhi, the translator of so much of the Buddhist canon, has put it, *lucid awareness.*[20] Easy to say. Not so easy to live.

When we take our seat in formal meditation, this intentional and embodied gesture of wakefulness and stillness in the posture we adopt is itself a radical act. In this fast-paced, twenty-four-seven, ever-connected, wireless world, getting people—especially Americans—to stop is revolutionary in and of itself. Then we can discover that stillness, coupled with wakefulness, is profoundly healing. Just to stop, to drop into the present moment, and to gently hold in awareness *whatever* is already here—the good, the bad, and the ugly, the full catastrophe—because it is all already here—and see what happens when you welcome it into awareness is a huge statement of the richness and potential within the domain of being. You might discover multiple hidden dimensions within yourself. You will certainly not find a direct experience of this domain within some ancient text or in some statue, although texts and statues can and do point to it. Ultimately you will only find the universe of awareness and its virtues within yourself. What is more, it has always been here—to be dis-covered or re-covered. Sometimes we recognize it in the present moment. Sometimes we even call it "the present moment"; and sometimes we call it "stillness" or "silence" or simply "awareness." Sometimes it manifests as stillness or wakefulness in motion. Whatever we call it, there are times when it hardly seems available to us, so lost do we get in all of our doing and thinking and reacting. The question is, Can the richness and depth of these aspects of our own being, these all-too-often hidden dimensions of being, be nurtured? And if so, then how do we nurture them?

The answer is "yes." We can indeed discover and nurture these hidden dimensions of our own being. And we do so through a certain kind of discipline. Through ongoing cultivation (bhavana), we are exercising and growing muscles of attention, muscles of kindness, muscles of self-compassion, muscles of wisdom. It is an act of self-compassion to sit down, establish yourself in a dignified posture, and put out the welcome mat for things as they are, with no agenda other than to be awake. Especially when you do not want to, or are too busy. It is a radical act of sanity—and a radical act of love. Over time, people come to live their way into this way of being and understand it inwardly. It cannot be understood merely through thinking. It has to be lived, or it is not understood.

This radical gesture of presence, clarity, and love is the essence of mindfulness practice and of MBSR, MBCT, and the rest of the family of mindfulness-based interventions. When they are delivered with adequate mastery of the form, content, intention, and process of their respective curricula, there is general agreement among the founders of MBSR and MBCT that these programs are 90 to 95 percent the same. The content has to be somewhat different at different junctures in order to address the needs of particular groups of people, as with those wanting to reduce their risk of relapse into major depression. But the overriding format and essence of the curriculum are the same—and the meditation practices are also virtually the same. The most important thing is always that the entire curriculum be grounded in dharma—even though we do not use the word *dharma* at all in MBSR or MBCT. In its embodied expression, however, as presence, as openhearted spaciousness, as kindness, all anchored in the ongoing practice and dharma understanding of the instructor, it is universal. There is suffering. That is universal. And there is the potential for liberation, right here and right now. That is also universal. And so we roll up our sleeves and work with what is here.

If you plot the number of scientific papers that have the word *mindfulness* in the title since 1980, the line goes along at a very low level until about 1997 or 1998. Then it starts to climb. At the time of this writing, it is going increasingly exponential, almost straight up. What started out in the basement of the University of Massachusetts Medical Center as something that few knew or cared about—and if they had known about it, in all likelihood many would have considered it to be crazy—is now integrated into mainstream science and medicine to an astonishing extent.

It is notable that the worlds of medicine and health care and beyond have said "yes" to the cultivation of mindfulness in the ways that they have, and that so many distinguished scientists and top-notch graduate students are drawn to conducting basic and applied research in this area. That was what I was hoping for all along, since I myself was not trained as a psychologist or a neuroscientist or, for that matter, to be a researcher of people. I did my early research as a graduate student in molecular biology on viruses, genes, and bacteria. But I knew enough about the value of the confluence of science and dharma in my own life to believe from early on that if we were able to show that mindfulness really made a difference in people's lives in the face of stress, pain, and chronic illness, the potential benefits could be huge—ultimately extending far beyond medicine, health care, and psychology—and that the potential for fundamental discoveries about the mind-body connection and the human psyche, brain, and heart would present compelling areas for rigorous scientific research.

How, you may ask, did we get from those initial goings-on in a hospital basement to this accelerating, exponential curve of mindfulness research? By putting one foot in front of the other and trusting that if we worked with people in an authentic way aligned with what is deepest and best within them and deepest and most appropriate to their suffering within the dharma, and published our results in reputable scientific journals, others would take note and say, "This is worthy of further exploration." Indeed, it might also appeal to them as human beings, and as a way to unify divergent elements and interests in their own personal and professional lives.

In the early days, we published a series of papers that looked at the effects of MBSR training on patients with chronic pain for whom medicine effectively had nothing left to offer. They had been, as they say in medicine, "failures" to all the other treatments. We also did a study of people with the skin disease psoriasis, an uncontrolled cellular proliferation in the epidermis that is exacerbated by stress. It is not cancer, but it expresses similar cellular factors as those expressed in basal cell carcinoma, or skin cancer. There is no cure for psoriasis, but there is a treatment to make it better temporarily: ultraviolet light. If you live in Europe, you can go to the Dead Sea and lie in the sun, because the sunlight, including the UV rays, are filtered by an extra 1,300 feet of atmosphere, and so you will not burn as readily. Often the health insurance in Europe will cover the expense of the trip. But if you don't have that luxury, or the time to travel, you can go for treatment to a phototherapy clinic, where you stand in a circular light box and get radiated three times a week for very short but increasing periods of time, up to ten minutes or so. You wear black goggles and a pillowcase over your head to shield your eyes and face. It is not like being out in the sun for an hour. It is more like being in a toaster oven. It is very intense, and there are high dropout rates from the treatment.

Our study had its beginning when my dermatologist colleagues wondered whether I could teach their psoriasis patients to meditate so that they would be more relaxed in the light box and tolerate the treatments more, and therefore be less likely to discontinue their treatments. When I heard this, I thought, *Wait a minute! This is an incredible experimental setup for seeing whether meditative practices can influence a healing process that we can actually see and photograph, and then ultimately study, in principle down to the level of gene expression and cellular mechanisms of action.*

The way the word *healing* is used in the field of mainstream medicine makes a big difference in how it is received by physicians and scientists. Sometimes it is wiser not to use the term at all, given its New Age connotations. When it comes to the skin, however, such as in the case of people with psoriasis, it is easy to see whether it is clear or has the scaly patches characteristic of the condition. Everybody can agree that the skin has healed, and that it can be seen and documented reliably. So, in collaboration with our dermatology colleagues, we conducted a study, published in 1998, that showed that in a randomized trial, the skin of people who were standing in the light box and listening to a guided mindfulness meditation audio program while undergoing the UV light treatments cleared roughly four times faster than that of the nonmeditators, who were getting the ultraviolet light treatment without the guided meditation. I would love to see this study replicated and extended.[21] Now, fifteen years after the original study was published, there are many more tools for assessing what may be going on, including tools for exploring possible biological mechanisms at the molecular and cellular levels of the skin.

From a scientific point of view, there has never been a better time to study the mind-body connection. In the past fifteen years, the science has changed so much that we have already had three remarkable, even revolutionary, methodological and conceptual advances. The first is the discovery of *neuroplasticity*, that the brain is continually reshaping itself in relationship to experience. Central to this is repetitive experience, which drives the neural changes. We know that there are certain regions of the brain, such as the hippocampus, important for learning and memory, where new functional neurons are laid down right up until the day we die. The old dogma was that from the age of about two, it was downhill in the central nervous system and that you lost neurons at an ever-increasing rate. In fact, the brain can remain dynamical throughout life and has the ability to recruit and repurpose more brain tissue (sometimes referred to as "real estate") for specific functions when the brain's activity is driven by and responding to specific and highly repetitive experiences. Trauma can degrade not just function but also the structure of the brain. But repetitive practices such as running, swimming, or meditation can actually refine and enhance the structure of the brain in the particular regions related to the nature of the experiences. With new developments in scanning technologies, there are now vastly improved tools for conducting these kinds of studies. Although they do not tell us everything about the brain or experience, they are windows into exploring the mind-body interface in new ways and coming to understand how such changes might be regulated by specific lifestyle choices. Recent studies from Sara Lazar's lab have shown that eight weeks of MBSR training can affect the gray matter density in a large number of regions in the brain that are essential for attention, emotion regulation, learning, and memory, thickening it in regions such as the hippocampus and thinning it in the amygdala.[22]

Another revolution in science has been the advent of the field of *epigenetics*. Epigenetics is based on the finding that there can be changes at the level of the chromosomes that influence gene expression without changing the genes themselves. In the old days we were taught that whatever genes we got from our parents, that was it, our genetic fate was determined. But it turns out now that our chromosomes are very dynamic structures, and how we live our lives can influence which of our genes get read or, in more technical terms, get expressed. For example, how you behave, or even what you eat, can turn on—the technical language is *up-regulate*—hundreds of genes and down-regulate hundreds of others. This is significant because many genes are linked to cancer. These are called proto-oncogenes. There are also pro-inflammatory genes. Neither of these types of genes does good things for the body when their expression is disregulated. The evidence is growing that when you take care of yourself in a certain way, including by enacting compassionate presence, you are selecting—not consciously of course—which genes are functioning and which genes are being quiet.

The third revolution is in the study of *telomeres* and the enzyme *telomerase*, work for which Elizabeth Blackburn at the University of California, San Francisco, shared the Nobel Prize in Physiology or Medicine in 2009. Telomeres are the long stretches of repeat subunits of DNA at the tips of all of our chromosomes. These degrade over time, with repeated cell division, but are repaired by telomerase. Chronic stress accelerates the shortening of the telomeres and thus accelerates cellular aging, because once the telomeres are gone, our cells go into senescence. However, the stress and shortening of the telomeres are mitigated by how stress is perceived. This suggests that if you practice transforming your relationship to stress, it could actually slow the aging process at a cellular level. A great deal of work is being done in this area (see chapter 4).

In another important advance within the growing field of mindfulness research, progress has been made in designing appropriate control conditions so we can be sure that the results we obtain are specific to the meditation practice itself. Richard Davidson and his colleagues at the Center for Investigating Healthy Minds at the University of Wisconsin have conducted a number of interesting studies recently using a control group called the Health Enhancement Program (HEP), designed specifically to match MBSR in all ways except for the incorporation of mindfulness practices. In a randomized trial of neurogenic inflammation in response to application of a skin irritant (capsaicin) to the forearm, Melissa Rosenkranz, Richard Davidson, and their colleagues have shown that while all self-reported changes in psychological distress and physical symptoms in response to a stress challenge were identical among members of the MBSR group and the HEP group, the MBSR group showed a significantly smaller post-stress inflammatory response than the HEP controls.[23]

I also want to highlight a study that Norman Farb, Zindel Segal, and their colleagues at the University of Toronto did with MBSR, looking at what they call different modes of self-referencing. They discovered that people taking the MBSR program showed reduced activity in a particular network within the frontal cortex of the brain—a midline network known as the default network—compared with controls. This network, which they term the "narrative focus" network, was also uncoupled from activity in a more lateral network, the "experiential focus" network, which showed greater activation after MBSR training and which is associated with moment-to-moment direct somatic experiencing. The narrative network can be thought of as a region that has a great deal to do with what we might call "the story of me and what is happening to me." The lateral region, especially on the right side, is more about direct somatic experience in the present moment—it is just mindful, with no story, more embodied. These results suggest that it is possible to learn, through the cultivation of mindfulness, to damp down somewhat on the "story of me" and to have a *decentered* perspective on it, in other words, a way of holding it in awareness without judgment but with discernment. It will still be here, and of course it is critical for us to be able to construct such narratives and for the mind to wander freely and unimpeded at times. That is in part the basis of our creativity and capacity for imagination. But it is important to develop in parallel other capacities within ourselves, in this case embodied present-moment awareness, and thus to mindfully exercise a flexibility of perspective so as not to be trapped in necessarily believing our internal narratives.

The Buddha is famous for saying that his entire teaching could be encapsulated in one sentence, "Nothing is to be clung to as 'I,' 'me,' or 'mine.'" As we have seen, neuroscientists are now identifying and studying various cortical networks that involve different modes of self-referencing. Further work along these lines may contribute in significant ways to elucidating important features of what we call "the self," a core question in the field of psychology. We thus have an extraordinary opportunity, at the confluence of these two epistemologies that have such different perspectives on the nature of self and different methods of empirical investigation, to ask important questions and design novel experiments to carry the field into new domains of insight. If we do not lose sight of the dimensions of dharma underlying meditative practices such as those integral to MBSR, this convergence has the potential to transform the science of the mind, transform the field of psychology, and transform the field of medicine. It will inevitably make health care a lot less expensive too, because we now have effective ways to motivate people to participate in their own health and well-being. This was the case in the psoriasis study, because the people in the meditation group healed faster and therefore needed fewer treatments to reach skin clearing. We have begun calling this approach "participatory medicine."[24]

The potential for us to transform the world both individually and collectively in ways that it is crying out for is enormous.[25] Transformation requires authenticity and creativity. No one can tell another person exactly how to go about it. But the invitation for all of us to inquire deeply along both first-person* and third-person† lines in this regard is itself a gateway to clarity, wise action, and well-being—for ourselves and for the world.[26]

---

* What we can learn through our own direct experience.

† What we can learn from the observed behavior and reported experience of others.

8

Therapeutic Applications of Meditation

Mindfulness-Based Stress Reduction

Dr. Edel Maex

Are thoughts dangerous, or totally harmless? In this chapter, Edel Maex, a pioneer of mindfulness training in Belgium, offers a glimpse of what it's like to take part in a Mindfulness-Based Stress Reduction class. He begins with a guided meditation designed to make us more aware of our thought processes, and the automatic patterns that can lead to worry, stress, and depression. When our thoughts are less solid and emotionally charged, he explains, healing becomes possible.

To give you a taste of what we do in mindfulness training, I will begin with a short guided meditation.

Please sit comfortably. If you like, you can close your eyes, or you can leave them open.

Start by bringing your attention gently to your breathing. Just be aware of the breathing in and the breathing out. Do not interfere with it. Do not meddle with it at all. Just leave it exactly as it is.

You may find that your breathing is regular and calm. If it is, just notice that. It is equally possible that you will find your respiration is hectic and irregular. Do not try to control it, but with kind, open attention, just notice that.

When you find that you have become distracted, and that your mind has wandered off, just let go of whatever caught your attention and return to your breath. Do that with kindness, because as you will notice, you have no control of the moment when your mind wanders off. The only control you have is to come back, so that is what you do. If thoughts or other things distract you, just notice, let go of them, and come back to your breathing.

As a next step, bring your attention to your thoughts, to what happens in your thinking mind. Notice the arising of your thoughts, and if something else distracts you, like your breath, for example, bring your attention back to this coming and going of thoughts. It is important to know that you are not your thoughts. Thoughts are just things that happen, so notice how a thought comes up, flowers, and, at a certain moment, is gone.

There might immediately be a next thought, or there might be a gap in between. Just notice for yourself how these things work, and do that with kind, open attention. By "open" I mean that you give equal attention to whatever thought arises, whether it is a pleasant thought or an unpleasant thought. Do not try to push away the unpleasant thoughts, and do not try to hold on to the pleasant thoughts. It is important to do this with a lot of kindness because you need that kindness, especially when unpleasant thoughts arise, in order to be able to stay with them and to watch it all happen.

The moment you get carried away and get lost in your

thoughts, just notice and, with kindness, return. You could start by coming back to the breath, and then return to watching your thoughts. You might have very smart thoughts, and you might have ones that are less smart. You might have thoughts that feel very much like they are coming from you, and you might have others that you do not understand why such things could happen in your mind. But with limitless kindness, just allow these thoughts to happen, and watch.

It is also helpful to be aware that you have no way of knowing what the next thought is going to be, so you can allow yourself not to know, and just look to see what happens, with a kind, open awareness.

Now you can open your eyes, if you had them closed, and start to move again.

Usually, when I do this in the hospital as part of an eight-week mindfulness training program, it is embedded in a longer guided meditation of about forty-five minutes. This particular meditation comes around the middle part of the course, in session five. Afterward I ask the group to split into smaller groups, I offer them some coffee, tea, and cookies, and everyone is given the opportunity to discuss their experience. After twenty minutes they come back and I ask them, "Well, how did that go?" One of the first things that always comes up is that some people—not everybody but many people—had the experience that suddenly there were no more thoughts. There you are, thinking that your thoughts are bothering you twenty-four hours a day, and then someone comes and tells you, "Just look at your thoughts." You shine your light on them, and *pff*, no more thoughts! It is very strange, but it shows us something about our thinking process. We think it is continuous, but it is not continuous at all—there are gaps between the thoughts. If I say to you, "Look over there!" you will look, and in that moment your thinking process will suspend. You will be open, looking, expecting, and receptive, and then it will start all over again.

Suppose you could live like that all the time, with the same continuous openness and receptiveness. When you apply that to the thinking process itself, then you notice that thoughts come and go, and there is an openness in between. In that moment, for a fraction of time, there are no more thoughts. Then the next thought is, *Hey, where are my thoughts?* The problem is that when people realize this, they think, *Now I know how it works. Now I know how to get rid of all my annoying thoughts. The next time I have a problem, I will sit and meditate all these thoughts away.* When you do that, you are in fact doing exactly the opposite of what you just did in the meditation, because now you are deliberately trying to get rid of your thoughts. It's a pity, but that is not the way it works.

As a next step in the training, I ask, "Exactly what is thinking?" At that point I speak for myself, because I cannot speak for the group. To be honest, when I do this practice and I watch the coming and going of my thoughts, I have to admit that the vast majority of thoughts that come up are pure nonsense. Maybe that is not how you experience it, but that is the way it works for me. That is how our minds work. The mind does exactly what it is supposed to do, and produces thoughts over and over and over again. This process is not completely random. There are some associative processes involved. When I think of the number one, for example, I think of two; and when I think of black, I think of white. But there is an array of thoughts that make me creative, and the more there are, the more creativity I can have.

Thinking is a process of selection. In this wild, flowering field of thoughts, I select which thoughts I want to continue with, and which ones I want to use. That is a very important thing to realize because very often we react to our thoughts automatically and we go with them, instead of responding consciously, instead of exercising the freedom that we have to choose what to do with our thoughts.

For example, whenever something happens, many people immediately have the thought, *Oh, it must be my fault.* Other people immediately think, *It must be someone else's fault.* People are different, but in the context of depression, it is usually the former. People think, *It's my fault.* These automatic thoughts come by themselves. I'm sure you are familiar with them. Some very popular ones are *It's my fault. I'm not good enough. I'm not worth it. Nobody loves me.* And they just keep coming. . . .

At first you are not even aware that these *are* thoughts. Nobody loves you, that is just how it is. You are not good enough, it is just a fact. But this exercise can help you to begin to realize that these automatically generated thoughts are always coming up. The moment you realize that you always have these thoughts, there is a moment where you say, *Oh, if only I could get rid of these thoughts. If only I could stop them*! Here's the bad news: you cannot stop them. This kind of thinking is too ingrained in our brain. There is too much "habit energy."

If you cannot stop these thoughts, then what can you do? You can become aware of them and exercise more freedom in how you deal with them. You can realize that the same thought keeps coming up, *I'm not good enough.* Even though you no longer want to have the thought, it is there. You cannot push it away, so what do you do? You invite it in, give it a place at the table, give it a cup of coffee, and just let it sit there.

To take a simple example, suppose you have your coat in your hands, you are just about to go outside, and a thought comes, *Nobody loves me.* You might react by hanging up your coat and lying back down on the couch. Another response might be just to notice, *Oh, no, there's that thought again. I wish I didn't have it, but I do. All the same, I'll put on my coat and go out and visit someone.*

One of the things that mindfulness practice teaches you is to watch your thoughts, to become aware of this dynamic, and to allow yourself for a moment not to react to thoughts but consciously, intentionally, just to watch what happens without acting on them. After all, thoughts are completely harmless! What could be less harmful than a thought? When I say that in my group, people start to protest. They say, "Thoughts are very dangerous!" In a way, yes, they are. Look at the major problems in the world. There are so many places where warfare and all sorts of terrible things are going on. Very often, wars are about thought. People are killed because of thoughts. Here I am telling you that thoughts are totally harmless, but when you turn on the television, you see that much bloodshed and so many problems are associated with thoughts.

When does a thought become dangerous? People sometimes say, "A thought becomes dangerous when you act on it." That is not strictly true. There is nothing wrong with a thought per se, and at a certain moment, you have to act on it. The fact that you are where you are now means that you have acted on some thoughts you had. A thought becomes dangerous the moment you make it solid, and you confuse it with reality. A thought becomes dangerous the moment you think, *That's the way it is. Anybody who thinks something different is wrong, and I will shoot him.* Sadly, that does happen. One of the most dangerous things that we can be in the world is "right." As long as I am wrong, there comes a moment when I stop. But when I think I am right, I do not stop. When you look at the places of conflict in the world, there are always two sides who both are sure they are "right." I once had a journalist in my group who had worked as a war correspondent, and she was devastated because she had friends on both sides of the conflict she was covering. She could understand that both sides, from their perspective, were right, and she could not cope with that. Being right is toxic for communication.

When I look more closely—say, for example, when I have an argument with my wife—what is usually the problem? We are both right! Is it only like that in my household, or do you recognize the pattern? If we want to move on from the argument, we have to make our thoughts fluid again. This might be simple to explain, but it is not so simple to do. What makes it so difficult is the emotion attached to the thought. All thoughts are emotionally laden. I used to think that we see something as true in the moment if it is logical, but it seems that this is not the way our brains work. We see something as true in the moment if it is emotionally laden. I'm a psychiatrist, and sometimes I see people with paranoia. Delusions are never emotionally neutral; they are laden with very strong emotions. The strength of our emotions makes it so difficult for us to let go of our thoughts.

In my experience, healing comes down to this process of mindfulness, where we look at our feelings in the same way we look at our thoughts—by not suppressing them, not losing ourselves in them, and by going with that middle way between ignoring and being carried away. It is in that moment that the healing of the emotion takes place.

This is exactly the same mechanism that people like Mark Williams, Zindel Segal, and John Teasdale looked to as a way of healing in depression when they developed the program that is known today as Mindfulness-Based Cognitive Therapy (MBCT). Depression is a mood disorder. A normal mood is fluctuating. We all have days when we wake up in the morning feeling like we can take on the world; and we have days when we wake up asking, *Do I really have to get up today*? That is a normal mood, it changes. Depression is the moment when your moods stop moving, when you are down and you stay down, for hours, days, weeks, or months. There is this downward spiral with very little oscillation, and it is terrible. When you are cured of depression, you return to normal. Your moods start oscillating again.

When you are down, quite understandably, you panic. *Oh, my god! I'm not going to be depressed again, am I? Tell me it's not true!* You wake up in the morning and say, *Oh no! Please! No depression! Not again!* You respond by trying to ignore it and push it away. *By noon it will be over. Try to ignore it!* With some luck, by noon it will be over. But if you are not so lucky, the panic, the fear, the whole process can start the cascade, revive the depressive process, and bring it back all over again.

What we learn in mindfulness training is to *see* a bad moment, a bad day, or negative thoughts and feelings—not to ignore them but to allow them to be there. You allow yourself to have a really bad day, maybe even a bad week or a bad month. You simply allow it to be there but without letting yourself get completely carried away by it. You stay in that open space, in that middle way between ignoring it and being carried away by it. That is what people learn to do. Then, even when they relapse into depression, they do it differently. Recently one lady said to me, "I got so much benefit from the mindfulness training. I'm so happy I did it, even though it didn't prevent my depression. But *now*, when I'm depressed, I'm able to look at it and deal with it differently." So it *did* help after all! When I mention the "middle way," which must sound familiar in a Buddhist context, the distance between the two pitfalls of ignoring and of being carried away is very narrow. But this middle way itself is very open. There is a lot of room in the middle way.

This is just a taste of how we do it in the mindfulness training, but there is one more thing to add, which I became aware of only recently. Some time ago, at a callback day for one of our groups, someone told me that before the eight-week program he had no problem at all with, say, killing a spider. But he had realized that now—and he did not understand why—he had difficulty killing a spider. When I asked the others, many people had experienced the same thing. In Mahayana Buddhism we are practicing in order to benefit all sentient beings. When people come to the hospital for mindfulness training, they do not come in order to save all sentient beings. They come for themselves, in order to deal with their own suffering. But many people discover that, in this open space, compassion seems to arise naturally, even though we do not explicitly speak about it in the classes. This is not a belief; it is something that you discover for yourself. It is not even logical, but it seems that when the human mind is open, compassion is the most natural thing to arise, and I think that is a key part of what we call mindfulness training.

9

Mindfulness in the Treatment of Depression

Observations of a "Decentered" Clinician

Dr. Lucio Bizzini

Over the past ten years, Mindfulness-Based Cognitive Therapy has emerged as a powerful ally in the battle against depression. Lucio Bizzini, who leads MBCT groups in Switzerland, explains how the program combines meditation with elements of cognitive therapy to help patients avoid being swept into a downward spiral of depressive thoughts. The result is a method that has been shown to halve the risk of relapse for people who have already suffered several episodes of depression.

As I prepared my presentation for the Meditation and Health conference, it was natural for me to look back at how I came to run mindfulness-based groups designed to prevent people from relapsing into depression. The first clue lies in the two main types of training I received, Piagetian psychology and cognitive behavioral therapy (CBT), in both of which the idea of *decentering* is fundamental. Jean Piaget wrote that "the most profound tendency of all human activity is progression toward equilibrium." Piaget's "genetic psychology" describes a gradual progression from the egocentric perspective of the infant to the decentered outlook of the young adult. This sense of "progressive equilibrium," or the gradual mastery of the human ability to accommodate different points of view, is very close to the idea of *taking distance*, which is one of the central characteristics of mindfulness.

Working in a psychiatric setting, I quickly became interested in the treatment of depression and I trained in psychotherapy, with a focus on CBT. In the treatment of depression proposed by Aaron Beck, a pioneer of CBT, there are several elements that dovetail closely with the Piagetian theory of decentering.[1] Indeed, one of the most effective therapeutic strategies for treating depressive patients is "cognitive restructuring," which is intended to modify, or at least soften, the content of depressive thoughts. This is achieved by helping patients gradually to become aware of these thoughts, and then to distance themselves from their negative content. Through self-observation during periods of sadness, irritation, or anger, the patient is helped by the CBT therapist to identify the "automatic thoughts" that give rise to depression, and to question or to modify certain assumptions or beliefs, which often turn out to be dysfunctional and only serve to sustain the depression.

At a later stage of therapy, the patient comes to recognize early patterns of maladjustment, developed during difficult events in life such as adverse emotional circumstances or periods of particular stress, that have led to depression. In some cases, the therapist and patient are able to work together to identify and then restructure these patterns. In other cases, the patterns can be looked at as hypotheses, rather than truths. This work is all about decentering and establishing distance from one's negative ideas about oneself, the world, or the future, which Beck identified as being at the heart of the depressive's thinking. Distancing oneself from one's thoughts, disidentifying oneself from them, and seeing them as mental events rather than as facts, theories about oneself rather than truths, are powerful means of getting out of depression. In CBT, working on the depressive aspects of thought is essential. It is one of the most effective tools for tackling sad moods and negative self-image, and is a key element in the cure of the depressed patient. This cognitive work, together with strategies of "behavioral activation," is still the preferred psychological treatment for depression.[2]

In the late 1980s, I was keen to deepen my knowledge of CBT, so I spent several months with colleagues at the Cognitive Behavior Therapy Unit at the Clarke Institute in Toronto. The unit's directors, the psychologists Jeremy Safran and Zindel Segal, were about to publish a book entitled *Interpersonal Processes in Cognitive Therapy*, in which the idea of decentering featured prominently. For the authors, decentering "is a process through which one is able to step outside of one's immediate experience, thereby changing the very nature of that experience. This process allows for the introduction of a gap between the event and one's reaction to that event. . . . Meditation is used specifically for the purpose of helping the student to obtain an experiential realization of the role that his or her own mind plays in constructing reality."[3]

Thus the link between decentering and meditation had already appeared in this work, well before the publication in 2002 of *Mindfulness-Based Cognitive Therapy*, by Zindel Segal, John Teasdale, and Mark Williams, and Jeremy Safran's *Psychoanalysis and Buddhism* in 2003.[4]

Back in Geneva, I worked with my colleagues at the Unit of Cognitive Therapy for the Elderly to set up a group therapy program based on Cognitive Therapy with Decentering Strategy (CTDS). The program, consisting of sixteen sessions, aimed at promoting decentering as a therapeutic strategy for treating depression in the elderly. The basic premise was that a depressive person who has an egocentric, negative vision of the world (somewhat disorganized and unnuanced, as Piaget might describe it) could draw upon his or her ability to decenter, built up over the course of a lifetime, in order to emerge from depression. In other words, you call upon your ability to imagine how it is to be in another person's shoes, to accommodate different points of view, to distance yourself from your own thoughts, and to observe your own behavior, in order to reduce the impact of depression.

The first component of CTDS is the classic CBT method of using self-observation and investigation of one's thoughts and emotions, as well as behavioral activation with a specific personal goal as the focus. The second component encourages decentering as a way for the depressive patient to achieve distance from his or her toxic thoughts and beliefs. For this we needed other strategies that were more experiential and more challenging, you could say. Here are three that we devised.

The first is a classic CBT approach that we called "putting yourself in the other person's place," which is done as a role-play. The second was inspired by an experiment devised by Jean Piaget and Bärbel Inhelder called "rotation of landscapes," which aims to develop one's ability to examine a situation from different points of view. We used the metaphor of a stone, which we invited people to examine from different angles.[5] The third method was suggested to us by Zindel Segal, and we called it the "strawberry effect." Jon Kabat-Zinn, taking his inspiration from the Buddhist teachings, calls it the "raisin exercise"; it is the first meditation exercise on his Mindfulness-Based Stress Reduction (MBSR) program.[6] In our CTDS manual, we described it as follows: "When we do something, we do it fully, taking notice of the different experiences and sensations involved. In other words, when we give something our full attention we can cut the flow of our discursive thinking and rumination."[7] In their MBCT manual, Segal, Williams, and Teasdale point out that the raisin exercise opens up new possibilities for experiencing something in a way that is quite different from what we are used to.[8] To conclude, this exercise illustrates Jon Kabat-Zinn's definition of mindfulness: "The awareness that arises by paying attention on purpose, in the present moment, and nonjudgmentally."

For the record, CTDS was not followed up, because the Unit of Cognitive Therapy for the Elderly closed in 2000 and I returned to the University Hospitals of Geneva to work on their newly created program for treating depression.

In August 2002, together with about thirty other clinicians, I took part in the first retreat organized by the creators of Mindfulness-Based Cognitive Therapy and Jon Kabat-Zinn. Not only was this crucial for my understanding of the underlying principles of mindfulness training; it was also, above all, a strong reminder of how important it is for the instructor to have his or her own personal meditation practice. Subsequently, I teamed up with colleagues in Geneva who specialized in the psychological management of mood disorders, and we ran the program twice more, while keeping up our regular personal meditation practices.

Convinced of the benefits of offering these mindfulness practices to our patients as a set of tools for regulating the emotions, we developed MBCT for use in our clinical practice, in both teaching and research.[9] As Pierre Philippot and Zindel Segal point out, research has shown that practicing mindfulness encourages a nonjudgmental, nonreactive attitude toward depressing thoughts.[10] It enables the patient to avoid reinforcing the content of these thoughts, and prevents him or her from being swept into a downward spiral of depression. There is a disengagement from the self-centered ruminations on all the whys and wherefores, causes and consequences. *Why? Why me? What's going to happen now?* Mindfulness brings nonjudgmental, nonreactive attention to bear on the present moment, and tumbling back into depression is averted.

Meditation practice is one way to promote decentering, by bringing us back to the present moment ("recentering" us) and by encouraging a benign curiosity and a letting go of our thoughts and emotions. It is a way of changing how we relate to our thoughts and emotions, a new attitude of welcoming the sort of difficulties in life that might put someone who has suffered from depression in the past at risk of relapse.

Mindfulness encourages a decentered relationship with mental content by giving people a wider perspective from which to observe their mode of thinking while their thoughts are unfolding. But how does a Mindfulness-Based Cognitive Therapy group actually work?

Once a patient is referred to us (usually this is a person currently in remission but with a history of depressive episodes, who has been referred by his doctor or psychologist), we see him once before the start of the group. We do a background check for suitability: past history of depression, level of motivation, availability for follow-up, and any contraindications such as substance abuse or trauma. Normally the group size is between eight and twelve members; there are eight sessions, and several follow-ups over the course of the year following the end of the program. All participants are offered the chance to practice together twice a week at lunchtime, and one evening every month.

As I give a brief overview of the eight-session program, it is worth bearing in mind that MBCT has been the subject of a number of controlled studies that have demonstrated its efficacy. The most recent replications show that MBCT delays relapse into depression, and halves the risk of relapse for patients in remission who have already gone through several depressive episodes.

Right from the start of the first session, participants are invited to discover a world based on experience and practice, using the raisin exercise mentioned earlier. The instructor places a raisin in the palm of each patient's hand, and invites the patient to look at it carefully, "as if you have never come across such an object before"—to examine its texture, shape, and so on. The exercise moves on quickly to the patients' being asked to be aware of any thoughts passing through their minds that draw them away from the object of mindfulness. Then they are asked to hold the raisin to their ear, to sniff it, to bring it to the mouth, put it in, chew it slowly, and swallow it with the deliberate intention of swallowing it. This experiment shows that when we begin to pay attention to things in a "fully mindful" way, our relationship to them changes. This is a powerful message, because it is easy to understand and based on personal experience. The participant develops an attitude of non-judgment, patience, and acceptance. There is a beginner's mind and a sense of letting go.

The group inquiry after we have done this exercise together is crucial in revealing the extent to which the instructor embodies the "mindfulness style" of being *inquisitive, kind*, and *confronting*. Inquisitive, because he or she encourages discovery: allowing ourselves to be surprised by this new way of relating to the things that go on around us, or in our minds. Kind, because the instructor reminds the participants of the importance of treating themselves with kindness—a radically different approach from the harsh and overambitious expectations that we often place upon ourselves. Confronting, because the instructor will gradually encourage the participants to welcome difficulties, to observe them, and not to fear them. The part played by the instructor, therefore, is crucial to the success of the program, but at the same time it is important to follow the MBCT manual as closely as possible. Systematic re-reading of the manual over the course of the program is strongly recommended for the instructor, as well as a thirty-minute period of preparation prior to each class. In our view, this is indispensable for creating an atmosphere that is immediately conducive to mindfulness.

In the first four sessions of the program, participants are introduced to a series of mindfulness practices such as meditation while lying down (also known as the body scan), sitting meditation, mindful walking, and stretching exercises (yoga). At the same time, participants are encouraged to incorporate mindfulness in their daily activities, and to develop their own personal "meditation program"—either sitting, lying down, or moving around, and with or without the assistance of a guided CD featuring the instructor's voice. A mini-meditation known as the "Three-Minute Breathing Space" is taught to help bring the practice of formal meditation into everyday life. In addition, MBCT incorporates certain exercises inspired by cognitive therapy, such as observing one's thoughts and feelings in a given situation, taking note of pleasant or unpleasant circumstances, and reading educational background material about the symptoms of one's condition. As in CBT, there are a number of specific exercises that are designed to be done at home.

These first few sessions encourage the participant to discover how useful it is to become more aware of his or her own body, and how the breath can be used to help us manage our emotions. This focus on the body is enhanced by varying the practices: the body scan brings out the link between boredom—fidgetiness—and the arising of negative thoughts. A long session of sitting meditation brings up the relationship between physical tension, pain, and the ability to recenter. The stretching exercises confront patients with their limits, and encourage a respect for the body. And finally, mindful walking reveals the wonderful richness of mindfulness, a faculty that we all possess but are not really aware of, and we are inspired to develop this further. All these discoveries, which are the result of direct experience, are discussed, brought into consciousness, and integrated into a new sort of knowledge: that the body can be a place from which to observe mental suffering, disengage from judgments and ruminations, and a space from which we can respond rather than react.

By the fourth session, it is time to confront the specific aspects of one's own personal territory of depression. This is the key moment in the program. The participant becomes aware that even if there is no depression around at the moment, danger lurks in the shape of old habits, which are never far away. The instructor can feel a change. The atmosphere, which up to now has been calm—lighthearted, even—darkens. The participants are aware that they are following the program because they have a high risk of relapse, especially those who have had several depressive episodes already. This is where the instructor brings kindness to bear, encouraging the patient to welcome difficult subjects and to find new routes out of the same old territory. Segal and his colleagues explain, "The aim of the fourth session is to explore how to 'stay present' in the face of the tendency to chase after the pleasant and avoid the unpleasant."[11]

We encourage the participants in the practice of equanimity, so that they neither grasp at happiness nor try to avoid difficulties. Rather, these are to be welcomed, observed, and their effects on the body experienced. This idea is illustrated beautifully in the poem "The Guest House," by the Persian Sufi poet Rumi, which we read in session five.[12] There is a long period of meditation, during which the difficulties faced by each participant are formulated and then shared. This is a way of checking whether or not the message has got through. Mindfulness practice does not lead to the practitioner embellishing things. Instead, its purpose is to develop in the practitioner a greater tolerance of unpleasant matters by becoming an inquisitive observer and asking, *What impact are these difficulties having on me?* This is a new way of allowing the experience to be: to look at it with curiosity and then let it go with a feeling of self-compassion.

Sessions four and five represent a transition toward learning the specific strategies that are used in the last three sessions. During moments of confrontation, it is helpful to recall these words from the manual: "Learning that we can actually stop struggling and be present gives us the opportunity to see and relate to our circumstances with greater clarity and directness."[13] The instructor will take more time during the sharing stages of sessions five and six to make sure he or she gets the message across.

The remaining sessions, particularly six and seven, are devoted primarily to various cognitive behavioral therapies. Session six concentrates on the work of distancing ourselves from our thoughts ("thoughts are not facts"). There are two approaches: we can work with thoughts as in the CBT approach—writing them down, changing the content, placing them in a wider context, and so on—or, with the help of the newfound strategy of mindfulness, we look at them, give them some space, and allow them to drift away like clouds in the sky or words on a cinema screen. In the CBT approach thoughts are restructured; in the second, we disidentify ourselves from them. This is a good illustration of how CBT has been developing recently.

The seventh session is called "How Can I Best Take Care of Myself?" We explore the link between mood and activity by identifying activities that lift your mood and those that dampen your mood. The idea is not so much to increase the kind of activities that energize us as to become more aware of them, so that we can anticipate moments when there is a dampening of mood. The instructions here become more specific: first we take a breathing space, and then we decide what we are going to do, either to stay with the thoughts or "take some action." This is not an easy process, and taking a gentle approach is advisable.

In the eighth session, participants are invited to develop a "relapse prevention action plan." This is a time for looking back, appreciating both one's own efforts and those of the instructor, and having confidence that the new way of mindfulness will prevent any further relapse. One participant said, "The Mindfulness-Based Cognitive Therapy program has enabled me to live more serenely and contribute to my own well-being. It's important to be really vigilant every day, so you don't miss out on even a single moment of meditation." The last session is also the time when fears of another relapse into depression emerge. Accordingly, we offer four more sessions over the following year so we can continue to work together and monitor how each participant's remission is going.

Statements made by the few patients who have relapsed into depression show that MBCT did, nevertheless, change something. One said, "I don't fall back in the same way anymore. I have a conviction that I can get myself back out of it again, and I get going on my plan of action." Another said, "MBCT changes how I relate to my thoughts and actions, and builds up my hope that better days lie ahead."

These statements are in line with the findings of numerous studies that have appeared mainly over the past five years, which have studied the psychological mechanisms describing the progress of patients following MBCT. They cite attention regulation, cognitive reactivity, and metacognitive awareness, among other gains made by patients.[14] Other authors have wondered whether there is a connection between the number of hours spent in meditation practice, by both the patient and the instructor, and a successful outcome. Results are inconclusive: a study published in 2009 by Emily Lykins and Ruth Baer suggests that keeping up a formal meditation practice is important in the prevention of a relapse,[15] whereas for James Carmody, writing in an article published the same year, improving the capacity to redirect one's attention, for example, to the breath, is a more important part of learning mindfulness than the amount of meditation practice done.[16]

As for us, we have been able to establish that 40 percent of the participants in our MBCT groups are still practicing one year after the end of the program. The great majority of them report that they have changed the way they relate to their thoughts, which are now viewed as mental events, not facts. When depression does recur, they find that the metacognitive element is crucial in speeding up their recovery. This encourages us to continue offering MBCT, and to go on refining our understanding of what works for the great majority of our patients.

In the future, we should be able to further adapt MBCT for patients suffering from chronic depression, and those with bipolar disorder. Further research should also enable us to identify the characteristics of patients who will not respond to MBCT or who have a relapse after doing the program. Other studies will need to be done to better assess the impact of the instructor's personal meditation practice on the overall success of MBCT groups.

I feel that this account of my journey as a Piagetian psychologist trained in cognitive behavioral therapy and mindfulness practices is now coherent and decentered. It seems to me that I have applied Piaget's principle of progression toward equilibrium, combining this with scientific knowledge and going beyond certain philosophical positions that are sometimes remote, if not contradictory. This is thanks to Piaget's famous ability to accommodate different points of view in psychotherapy, something he always practiced. It is this vision of being decentered that has easily enabled me to bring together standard methods of CBT with treatments based on mindfulness, cognitive restructuring, and disidentification from one's thoughts. There is only one requirement for this practice of "progressive equilibrium": do it with kindness.[17]

10

Mindfulness in a Palliative-Care Setting

Ursula Bates

Is there a place for meditation in the care of terminally ill patients? The clinical psychologist Ursula Bates shares her experiences of running a mindfulness program at a hospice in Ireland. She describes the adaptations made to accommodate frail patients and the basic exercises, such as "grounding practice," that they can use to support themselves. The voices of the patients provide a moving testimony of the challenges they face, the strength they draw from being part of a group, and the ways mindfulness helps them as they approach the end of their lives.

Core values support any work in end-of-life care, and mindfulness holds that each individual has inner resources that can be aroused to support coping and reduce suffering. Quality of life is a worthwhile goal when active treatment and cure are no longer options, and this includes physical, emotional, spiritual, and existential domains, both for the patient and for caregivers and family members. A good death in palliative medicine is a death as pain-free as possible, in the place of one's choice, accompanied by one's loved ones. But above all, the overriding philosophy of Dame Cicely Saunders, the founder of the modern hospice movement, is treasured by all who work in this field: "You matter because you are you, and you matter to the end of your life. We will do all we can, not only to help you die peacefully but also to live until you die."

Background

Blackrock Hospice serves a catchment area of 250,000 people in South Dublin, Ireland, providing a home-care, day hospice, and inpatient service. It is a publicly funded service, providing equal access for people from all cultural and religious groups. The day hospice opens three days a week, from 10 A.M. to 3 P.M. Patients receive nursing care, physiotherapy, hydrotherapy, and complementary therapy, and they and their families have the option of attending the social work and psychological service.

Our patients have a wide variety of metastatic malignant and nonmalignant terminal conditions. All have been referred by their general practitioner or medical consultant, and have been informed of their transition from curative to supportive care. Their level of insight varies, and it is common for patients to fluctuate in their capacity to acknowledge their limited prognosis. The patients have a wide range of physical disabilities and vulnerabilities: they are coping with the residual effect of chemotherapy, operation sites, scar tissue, and a limited range of limb mobility, and they are at risk of spinal cord compressions and falls.

On assessment, most patients are offered the opportunity to attend classes in Mindfulness-Based Stress Management, an adapted version of Jon Kabat-Zinn's Mindfulness-Based Stress Reduction (MBSR) program. They are encouraged to attend one taster session and then to withdraw if they are not comfortable with the class, because their capacity to manage in a group is the most important consideration. This inclusive system has led to a good ongoing attendance by male patients, who are generally slow to avail themselves of therapy services. A small number of people have been excluded since the classes started in 2006, mainly because of serious agitation, moderate to severe hearing loss, or ongoing serious psychiatric difficulties. Patients who have moderate to severe post-traumatic stress, clinical depression, panic disorder, and organic conditions are assessed and treated individually and then, if appropriate, referred to the mindfulness group.

Palliative patients are all different in the way they react to this critical life transition, as the following two examples demonstrate. In the first case, Andrew left the group despite having all the psychological skills needed to participate, whereas for John, although he had limited skills, mindfulness became a significant part of his journey.

Andrew, fifty-one, was a recently diagnosed multiple sclerosis patient who joined the mindfulness group and found it emotionally overwhelming. He was tearful afterward, as he had not spoken openly about his deterioration and found that when he engaged with the breathing exercises he was engulfed by his own unexpressed grief. He was referred to individual counseling on the understanding that he could rejoin the group once he felt able to engage with the work.

John, forty-three, had multiple myeloma. A single man, living alone and with limited social contacts, he was very reserved and initially refused all services. Having been referred by the nurse manager for individual assessment, he revealed a lifelong history of social anxiety and withdrawal. He had difficulty with his diagnosis and a very limited ability to explore his emotional life. He was encouraged to try mindfulness for a few sessions, and was assigned an individual counselor for supportive work. He attended the day hospice for over a year and was always a quiet but attentive group member. He came to the ward for his final weeks and used the body scan and mindful breathing techniques right up to the end of his life.

Getting Started

The mindfulness group meets each morning and is open to all patients. Group sessions are forty-five minutes long, so over a twelve-week period a patient will receive nine hours of mindfulness, which is the equivalent of about one-third of the teaching of a standard eight-week MBSR course. The groups are open, and patients come once a week for twelve weeks, with the option of continuing for a further twelve weeks if they feel it will be of benefit. Most choose to stay for twenty-four weeks, so they receive a total of about eighteen hours of group work. Given these constraints, the overall aim is to introduce the patients to mindfulness, to establish a short breathing practice, support their capacity to sit for fifteen minutes, reconnect them to their bodies, and develop an orientation toward acceptance of the "here and now." All groups are taught by an experienced mindfulness teacher and attended by the psychology interns at the hospice.

The groups meet in a bright room facing the garden, and the patients are seated in supportive chairs. Only very gentle upper body stretching can be included in the mindfulness classes because of the physical limitations of the patients. Interruptions, while kept to a minimum, have to be tolerated as patients occasionally need to leave the group for individual appointments. It is best to include such movement and noise from a busy unit in the exercises right from the beginning, rather than its later becoming a source of irritation.

Before the start of the class, the nurse manager will update the mindfulness teacher on the attendance, absences, and physical difficulties of the patients who will be attending on that day. If a patient has died since the previous week's class, we will include a reflective session in which we may light a candle, dedicate the breathing exercise for the benefit of that person, and spend some time recalling memories of their time with the group. At the time of this writing, the Wednesday group has four robust members who have now attended six classes. They are highly motivated to engage and can sustain a fifteen-minute guided breathing exercise. Two others have just joined, and one of them is quiet and disengaged.

The Power of Intention

Many of the patients who come to our day hospice have not specifically committed to attending a mindfulness program. When we ask people to be present and aware in a hospice setting, therefore, we are often asking them to effect a radical reorientation of their own state of mind. In my teaching, I think of this as calling to an emergent potential that people themselves may not be aware of consciously but that is present nevertheless.

As I sit in the day room, I see around me people with ambivalent or mixed intentions, who have the potential to move in the direction of mindfulness but do not yet have any conscious awareness of what they desire or what might unfold. I begin therefore by asking them to consider choosing to be here, in this place, at this time, together. This brings up anger and bitterness, as well as acceptance and resignation. Questions such as *Why me?* are aired and discussed by members of the group. Stories emerge of being sent to the hospice by medical professionals, feelings of being abandoned by professionals and family members, and the sad feeling of being a burden. All are named, shared, and accepted. Jon Kabat-Zinn tells us that the attitude with which we undertake mindfulness practice can be compared to the soil. Good soil is loose, open, damp, and warm, full of a range of decaying matter and organisms. In our groups, this image deepens and returns again and again, as patients begin to find a place for "negative and disturbing emotions," which become manure and fertilizer for the soil.

In choosing to be present, some sense of freedom returns to many for whom their recent lives have been an experience of disempowerment. As each week passes, the choosing becomes more intentional, as people make the conscious decision to turn up for the work and to turn up to themselves, however they are in the moment. Courage deepens with each choice.

Grounding

Learning to be present requires palliative patients to engage with their bodies, and to turn toward an experience with which they have dissociated themselves in order to cope with medical investigations and treatment. Grounding is a step-by-step, sensory way to reengage, offering the mind a concrete anchor to support it in coming back into contact with the body. Patients with post-traumatic stress symptoms benefit from basic grounding to regain a sense of control. Grounding can also be applied easily to everyday situations that are stressful for patients, such as moving from sitting to standing, fear of falling, or episodes of anxiety. Repeatedly they describe a mind-body gap; although their experience of their mind and spirit is of being about thirty-five years old, they are constantly adjusting to living with a failing body. They anticipate moving as if they were younger and often find themselves losing their balance when they try to do so.

Patients share many difficulties, such as short-term memory issues and problems coping with daily activities, and using mindfulness to keep their full attention on the moment can help them discover ways to manage these difficulties. Through a compassionate attention to the needs of our bodies, an inner wisdom begins to emerge. For example, Carmel was distressed by the fact that she had lost her keys a number of times; she used the grounding exercise to steady her mind and support her memory. "I held the door keys in my hand and felt the metal and the coldness," she said. "Then I looked at the bowl in front of me, gently put the keys inside and focused on them in the bowl. I took a few slow breaths. The next morning when I woke up I could picture them in the bowl."

Here is a basic grounding practice:

Take a moment to settle yourself on your chair.

Close your eyes if that feels comfortable for you.

Notice where your feet are . . .

The point of contact between your feet and the ground . . .

Or your heels as they rest against the chair.

Moving your attention up your body, notice the gentle pressure of the chair against the back of your legs.

Bring your attention to that sensation. Notice the temperature of your legs, and the texture of your skirt or pants against your legs.

Moving your attention up along your back, feel the pressure of the chair against your back, the sensation of hotness or coldness, and the feeling of the fabric, rough or smooth.

Notice what your hands are touching. Feel the texture and temperature against your hands.

Gently take a moment to tune in to your body.

Do you notice any tension in your legs or back?

If you need to move any part of your body then do what you need to do, slowly and mindfully.

Gradually assume an upright and dignified posture.

Attention Practices

It takes effort to work with the energy in your mind and body, and mindfulness requires not just passive agreement but an active engagement, a conscious intention. Most patients are on medication for pain management, which dulls their acuity and induces periods of drowsiness. I frequently ask meditation practitioners who have been medically ill to talk to me about their experience of their formal meditation practice during illness. Most recall being unable to engage in formal practice and relying on short practices and external supports, such as pictures of a teacher, audio recordings, or simply resting in a sense of trust that others were practicing on their behalf.

With palliative patients, therefore, it is essential to have a range of objects on which to focus one's attention, and very small goals. In *The Tibetan Book of Living and Dying,* Sogyal Rinpoche cites three central meditation techniques that can be used as part of a simple practice: focusing on an object, reciting a mantra, and watching the breath.[1]

The awareness exercises that we teach in our mindfulness classes include focusing on an object in the room, such as a painting or a plant, or on an object in the garden. The patients can also focus on an "object in the mind," such as a safe place, or a loving friend or relative. There is also a mindful eating exercise that involves chewing a raisin, as well as the gradual body scan, gentle upper body stretching, and mindful breathing.

All patients must be able to sustain mindful breathing for at least a short period before they can move on to the last four sections of the eight-week MBSR course. Consequently, when a new member joins an established group, we have to move back to the beginning exercises. We describe this as going back to core practice and encouraging everyone to work at their own pace with their own internal world. Our experience is that with a steady, established group, the new member integrates and is supported by the depth of concentration in the others. With a weaker group, the teacher needs to take a more active and structured approach. While this constant shifting is not ideal for learning, it reflects the challenge of mindfulness—to use what is available here and now, even when it is far from perfect. It removes another layer of the standards we set for ourselves, of how, where, when, and with whom we can practice. It is important for the teacher to keep a record of the sessions, so there is a consistent teaching of the core attitudes even as the sessions flow back and forth through the eight-week course.

As a teacher I have to be mindful that members of the group sometimes fall asleep and to include it in the practice. In the group we speak of it as "going to and coming back" and we encourage a sense of flow with the experience. We strongly encourage people to notice, *Now I am drifting into sleep, and now I am coming back,* and to focus their awareness on the movement with gentle curiosity. As one approaches death, the mind will experience a range of different states—drifting, dreams, loss of clarity, and a gradual withdrawal from the world of phenomena—so the experience of working with the movement of these states is important both for the patients and for the teacher.

Gradually, there is a deepening trust that the group is a place where we can be both aware and unaware, and an ability to tolerate altered states while trusting that the inner self endures.

Sometimes it is necessary to support an agitated, deaf, or blind patient in the breathing practice. To do this, I will ask the main group to establish a mindful breathing practice and to continue to rest in that. I then ask the agitated patient to keep his or her eyes open and look at me, or at an object. I sit quietly and pace the patient's breath, breathing at the same pace and in the same place (upper chest, stomach, or lower stomach) as the patient is breathing. As I continue pacing, I will say, "On the next outbreath, I'm going to place my hand on your hand." Then, "On the next inbreath I'm going to gently squeeze your hand." I continue with the meditation and gently squeeze the patient's hand on each inbreath. As I am doing that, I gradually allow my own breathing to return to its normal pattern, very gently watching for any deepening or slowing in the breath of the patient, and pacing my hand movement to reflect this. Frequently the patient will gradually begin to match the breathing pattern of the group.[2]

Sharing within the Group

Mindfulness sessions are based on each group member keeping a focus on the sensory experience of the practice. Another vital element, however, is sharing, which plays a crucial role in building the culture of the group. Sharing within the group needs to be encouraged, as this is often the only space in which patients can talk about the daily difficulties and misunderstandings that are part of having a chronic illness.

Shemus, who had been so shocked by his palliative status that he had spent about six months in bed waiting in terror for death, often welcomed the new members into the group. He said once, "I thought I was dying. It took a respite stay on the ward [for things to change]. It was hard to come in. Festus [the physiotherapist] sat by my bed every day and gradually got me to walk. Then, coming to the group, I began to understand that I was experiencing panic attacks. I still get them now, but I can steady myself with the breathing and I can tell people around me what is happening. This is a place where you can talk about what is going on inside, and not take to the bed like I did."

Joe, seventy-six, spent a lot of the time in day hospice being tense and irritable. He attended the mindfulness group and for weeks would say to me, "Ursula, you're a nice girl, but you talk a load of rubbish." However, he did participate in all the exercises and gradually built up a genuine trust in the other group members. In his working life, he had been a senior bank official and run a large organization. He found his illness deeply distressing because it limited him to his home and the company of his wife, who was seriously mentally ill. One day he arrived quite agitated and reported, "I don't know what you're doing to me here! Last night I was watching the Angelus [a brief Catholic religious exercise which precedes the evening news on the main national television station in Ireland] and when the image of potato shoots growing came on, I suddenly found myself crying in front of the television." He started to cry again. The group, mostly men, said to him, "Now you're becoming one of us Joe. You're having feelings. What are those feelings exactly?" Joe said, "As I saw the potatoes, suddenly I was ten years old again, planting potatoes with my father in the west of Ireland." All of Joe's years of hard work and responsibility had fallen away and he was a boy once again, working the land with his father. That day we read Seamus Heaney's poem "Digging" in the group, and gradually his distress and tears reduced.

Joe's experience reminded me of Jon Kabat-Zinn's words about mindfulness practice: *You don't have to like it; you just have to do it.* From the doing, change begins.

Poetry and Stories

All our patients in palliative care have been journeying with a serious illness and many have been in very difficult medical situations. Caroline Garland, a specialist in the study of trauma, describes a traumatic event as "one which, for a particular individual, breaks through or overrides the discriminatory, filtering process, and overrides any temporary denial or patch up of the damage. The mind is flooded with a kind or degree of stimulation that is far more than it can make sense of or manage."[3]

Patients have subjective, internal experiences for which they often have no words. Poetry offers images and a language that awakens the imagination, from which a depth of understanding can begin to flow. Finding an image or expression of emotion that matches one's internal experience and allows it to be shared in the group enables the mind to digest the distressing material and reset its boundaries. Internally, the patient expands his or her capacity to bear difficult states. In his exploration of the poetic imagination, Gaston Bachelard speaks of the reverberations of even a single poetic image: "By its novelty, a poetic image sets in motion the entire linguistic mechanism. The poetic image places us at the origin of the speaking being."[4]

During one of our group sessions, a mute patient with oral cancer gestured excitedly when we read the following passage by Rainer Maria Rilke: "So you must not be frightened . . . if a sadness rises up before you larger than any you have ever seen; if a restiveness, like light and cloud-shadows, passes over your hands and over all that you do. You must think that something is happening with you. . . ."[5]

Pointing to herself, she wrote the word *sadness* on her notepad. Gesturing with her hands, she showed us a sadness bigger than herself. When we have a group of particularly elderly or cognitively fragile patients, we find that *Favourite Poems We Learned in School as Gaeilge*, by Thomas F. Walshe, can be a useful resource.[6] These poems, which many Irish children have learned by heart, remain with us until the end. In one group, Kitty, who was gently fading and could no longer read, was delighted to recite out loud "Trees" by Joyce Kilmer. To her great pleasure, the whole group joined in.

Building a Community

Irvin Yalom, in a seminal article in which he describes a four-year psychotherapy group for the terminally ill that he led, noted that the threat of death is such that "most psychotherapy patients and most therapists will not stare at death very long before they lower the blinds of denial." Yalom reported that the lesser dreads and losses are more often approached, such as separation, loss of sexuality, and the loss of ego boundaries. In the face of such anxiety, defenses such as denial, depression, and avoidance are activated. Already in 1976—before the development of mindfulness—Yalom was offering these patients meditation practice and pain management before the group sessions.

As curative factors in the group therapeutic process Yalom cites altruism, catharsis, group cohesiveness, universality, and existential factors. Mindfulness is a distinctly different method to psychotherapy, yet these factors are also relevant to facilitating the type of slow, open groups that are suitable for a day hospice setting. Their activation requires that time be given to group sharing and the naming of denied feelings such as despair and dread.[7] Siegfried Heinrich Foulkes, the founder of a type of group therapy called group analysis, has two useful concepts that support group work in this setting. One is that the group mind is fundamentally more robust and healthy than the individual mind. The second is that when the individual speaks in a group, he or she is often speaking on behalf of other members of the group, which allows the group leader or therapist to link comments by one group member to the concerns of another.

Pat, seventy-nine, is the primary caregiver for her husband, who has dementia. She was sent to a boarding school as a child, and has a particularly bitter and negative stance toward all treatment and medical settings. Initially she used the group to complain whenever possible about treatment and to denigrate the work. Drawing on my training in group analysis, I suggested to her that she was holding an angry position on behalf of the entire group and all women who were medically ill, and that she should continue to voice her rage. The group, mainly women, agreed with this. At times I would wonder aloud whether Pat was working too hard and maybe someone else would like to voice her anger. Gradually she participated more and it emerged that she had a deep love of poetry. She started reciting poems in the group and we sourced the poems and read them out together. She became an active group member and stayed in the day hospice for twenty-four weeks. Her anger diminished and, behind it, her profound loneliness emerged.

Catharsis is not directly encouraged or discouraged in mindfulness. As strong feelings arise, I simply support people in experiencing them in the moment, and as calmness returns, I try to explore where the feelings are held and name them. "So in your stomach there was a heavy feeling, and the word that comes to mind is 'despair.' How would it be to be present to it, soften toward it, and allow it space?"

Kindness for Oneself and Others

In line with Yalom's observations of his terminally ill psychotherapy groups, the patients in these groups are, in my experience, exceptionally cohesive and supportive of one another. I have been struck by how creative and sensitive they are in their support. Sensing Pat's isolation and her difficulties in being positive, group members spontaneously started bringing in little gifts for her—cards, images, poems, or small bouquets of garden flowers—to which she responded with a childlike delight. After week twenty-four, she requested to be allowed to stay on at day hospice.

Loving-kindness meditation is a gentle and useful practice with which to end a group session, as many patients need consistent support to treat themselves with compassion. After the loving-kindness practice, we close the session by dedicating what we have just done for the benefit of others. This is openly received by palliative patients, who are deeply motivated to be of use to others and frequently see themselves as a burden. It also relieves the worries they have about leaving family members who are perceived to be vulnerable. For example, Helen, who attends the Tuesday group, has a forty-year-old son with multiple sclerosis who lives in a care home. He is very emotionally dependent on her and calls her on the phone up to three times a day. She feels that she is the only one who understands him, and worries about how he will cope when she is gone. She dedicates her practice to him. (In May 2012, as I was editing this chapter, Helen died very peacefully on the inpatient ward. Her son had died the previous day in his care home.)

Frequently, the group members dedicate their practice to the other patients on the inpatient unit. This has a very tender benefit when, weeks later, a group member will find himself on the ward. When I visit and sit with him, he will know that the group is meeting in day hospice, practicing, and so the circle closes.

Research

Between 2008 and 2009, an independent research psychologist interviewed patients who had completed twelve weeks of the mindfulness program at the Blackrock Day Hospice, and used open questions and thematic analysis to evaluate the interview data. Seventy-three patients with advanced cancer had completed a combined total of 461 classes, and 66 agreed to be interviewed about their experience. The following themes were reported; the figures indicate how many of the 66 patients cited each theme:

Mood management	52
Normalization	52
Giving help	49
Nonjudgmental	45
Acceptance	43
Reducing isolation	41
Reducing ignorance	41
Openness	37
Common humanity	31

The sections that follow include quotations from the participants that communicate the different ways they felt the mindfulness program and the environment of the group had benefited them.

Mood Management

Fifty-two participants said that they had actively used the breathing exercises as a coping tool. Whereas previously they had felt helpless or ashamed in the face of their fragility, now they were aware, present, and able to respond to their daily struggles to cope physically and emotionally.

"If I catch myself becoming depressed, I try to do the breathing exercises and I notice that I feel less anxious and more relaxed."

—Carmel, forty-four

"I used to feel anxious all the time. I would rate my own anxiousness before the course as a ten, but now it's as low as a three."

—Tony, eighty-two

Normalization, Reducing Isolation, and Engaging with Common Humanity

The three factors of normalization, reducing isolation, and engaging with common humanity were woven through every interview. The relief experienced in sharing with others who were in a similar position was expressed by all.

"On each seat I could see a vision of myself." —Tony

"It legitimized my feelings of being sick, realizing that others were too, and that I didn't need to keep putting a brave face on things." —Shemus, sixty-nine

"I'm not so isolated now. I used to go from one week to the next without talking about cancer. I didn't care about anything before I went to the group. The group helped with this." —Joe, fifty-two

Reducing Ignorance

Initially, the participants in the mindfulness group were surprised by the emphasis on learning new ways of being. At a point where the social narrative seems to be about their being useless, and they have fears about the medical system giving up on them, we are presenting them with a challenging, active invitation to engage radically with their experience.

"Before I started the group I was constantly scared and frightened about my illness and believed it had the ability to attack at any time. I often got stressed about falling down dead on the street, or going insane and killing someone. With a combination of helpful information from the health staff at the hospice, giving me a full explanation of my illness, and using breathing, I have avoided such feelings of fear." —Carmel

Giving and Receiving Help

Participants spoke of the pleasure they experienced in being of assistance to others in the group, both by sharing and by supporting one another in the practice. They also talked about their own experiences of receiving help, and the struggles they faced in becoming more dependent on others and being open to allowing others to help them.

"I enjoyed helping others, still being of use." —Pat, seventy-nine

"Sometimes a stranger can open a door a family member can't, and correct you or give hope." —Tony

Acceptance

Many spoke of their struggle to accept where they were in their lives. The link between acceptance and the capacity to engage with and manage their daily lives had become clear for many. This level of acceptance is close to a sense of self-control and self-authoring.

"It helped me to lower my expectations—my physical expectations—and know my limitations." —Shemus

"It helped me come to terms with myself—to accept that my body is 'rotting away.' That brings it home why you are here. Once you come to terms with it, you can enjoy what you have left."
—John, forty-three

Openness

Often openness began externally, through communication in the group. Joe worked as a truck driver and came to the group on the understanding that he would not have to share if he did not want to. He was silent for about four weeks and eventually he began to talk. In his interview, he told us what had moved him. Later, that openness extended to family members and finally to his inner self.

"I surprised myself. Seeing others open up made it easier for me to do the same. It's not something that comes naturally to me. I normally play my cards close to my chest, but I saw there was no value to this and if no one spoke out, no one would benefit. In the last few weeks I have spoken a bit to my wife. She always wanted to talk, but I didn't, and the group helped with that. Now I can't stop."

Satisfaction Ratings

Seventy-three percent of the group members who were interviewed said they were satisfied or very satisfied with the program that we offered. The 21 percent who expressed moderate satisfaction had difficulties applying the method in their daily lives. They reported that they were able to use it in the group but had problems generalizing the learning outside. Low satisfaction was expressed by three people who did not like the method and found it hard to engage with.

"I was not aware of the fact that there was a support group like this. I thought you would have to be special to avail [yourself] of it. I do have faith in human nature, and it's good to know people care."

—Kitty, eighty-six

Reflections

Palliative care is a complex, specialized field for the application of psychological interventions and mindfulness interventions. Expectations of results have to be modified to reflect the declining physical and mental ability of patients. MBSR and MBCT are, in the format of the eight-week course, designed as a rigorous teaching that requires formal practice and integration of mindfulness into daily life. In palliative care, patients are learning in the face of a major life challenge, and they have limited energy for formal practice.

Our research, while exploratory, suggests that mindfulness is a useful method for the reduction of emotional distress, improving communication and coping skills, and reducing the isolation of palliative patients. Group satisfaction ratings were consistently high, and patients found the program to be accessible. In terms of health economics, the program does not reduce costs, as it requires considerable planning and follow-up, but it increases access and the use of psychological methods for male patients and the elderly population, both of whom underreport mental health issues and underuse psychological therapies.

When we compare the experience of our palliative mindfulness patients with the literature on models of mindfulness, several areas of similarity and difference emerge. The two defining factors of mindfulness cited by Scott Bishop, self-regulation and orientation toward experience, are evident in the data.[8] Patients reported better regulation of mood, increased communication both within and outside the group, and greater focus on and appreciation of the present, and some gained a more holistic sense of themselves. The majority of the participants felt a turning toward their experiences. They were more accepting of their illness and more connected to their physical and emotional states. For some this was fulfilling, and for others somewhat disturbing.

In our own work, we believe that there are four active movements toward reduced distress and a strengthened capacity to live with a chronic illness: intention, attention, turning toward the difficult, and kindness. *Intention* activates a sense of choice at a difficult time. Palliative patients come because the group is recommended to them and their active participation needs to be encouraged. This is echoed in the experience of the patient who came even though he did not know what to expect. The main intention voiced by people in the group was to help themselves to cope, not with death and dying but with living with limitations. *Attention*, which is the most actively taught skill, was used extensively by the group members as a coping tool. They all, in their own individual ways, *turned toward difficulty*, opening up, sharing, reducing avoidance, and replacing old stories and ruminations with new stories—some sadder, but all more connected. But it was *kindness* in all its manifestations that the group spoke about, and kindness they saw in each other's faces, brothers and sisters on the road, learning from each other, helping and allowing themselves to be helped.[9]

PART FOUR

Meditation and Spiritual Care

11

Using Meditation to Improve Standards of Care and "Well-Treatment"

Dr. Cathy Blanc

Is there something missing from the training that doctors, nurses, and other health-care professionals receive? Cathy Blanc thinks so, which is why she founded the Tonglen Association, a group of volunteers who teach meditation and other contemplative methods at medical institutions in France. Unless we know how to take care of ourselves, she writes, we will not be able to take care of others—and meditation is a key support that gives us the space and strength to respond to challenges in a different way.

How can we deal with all the suffering that we face in life, be it bereavement, separation, illness, dissatisfaction, and, of course, death? Not to mention the growing plague of Western illnesses such as depression and low self-esteem, which still seem to be relatively unknown in at least some parts of Asia. And how do we reconcile the demands of our high-tech society, as it attempts to push back the frontiers of illness and death, with the needs of our inner "self," which seeks ethical values, humanity, and simplicity? The answer is to be found in our ability to create an approach that I call "caring for oneself—caring for others." This is the life force of all care activity, and meditation is one of the tools, drawn from Buddhism, that enables us to put this dynamic relationship into practice. This back and forth between oneself and the other allows us to grow as human beings, and to act as if we are writing *Other* with a capital O. Meditation is a simple, powerful, and profound technique that helps us to face difficulties and gives us an opportunity to live better. It is an integral part of our approach to care, and we offer it to everyone.

In health care, *well-treatment* has become a central issue for patients and caregivers alike. It is an attitude that we need to learn and develop as an antidote to mistreatment. Mistreatment comes in many forms, can be active or passive, and is often brought on by the ignorance, unease, or fear that suffering and death can provoke in us. It is also linked to the attitudes and behavior that result from stress, the increasing pressure that is placed on health-care professionals, and the psychosocial risks that they face.

Rather than analyzing the causes of mistreatment in an attempt to find solutions to the problem, at the Tonglen Association we decided to turn our minds to developing a "well-treatment" approach toward both oneself and others. Whatever we are doing, whether it is providing care or training health professionals, our focus is always on the human aspect. How do we develop a quality of listening that will enable each of us to find the creativity and resources within ourselves to respond on this level?

The experiences that I am going to describe here are primarily based on caregiving. Since 1994 we have worked with people facing all kinds of difficulties, and our members have spent a lot of time at their side. In a universal, secular way, we share with them some of the priceless gems from the Buddhist teachings, because contained within these teachings are some extremely useful tools to help us find peace and serenity, and to face situations in a different way. These teachings provide a methodology, a know-how, and a science of mind that are simple to explain and to connect with our own reality. Everything is there. At the same time, I like to remind people that this richness and wisdom can be found in all the great spiritual and philosophical traditions, even if they are not structured and presented in the same way. The Tonglen Association was founded upon this very secular approach, and we have worked hard to try to draw out, hone, and clarify the Buddhist teachings and practices so that they can be shared with others in all their relevance, depth, and effectiveness.

The act of caring teaches us very quickly that the people we are caring for have a richness that we must discover if we really want to be able to help them, and to stop exhausting ourselves in the process. During their lives, these individuals have gathered knowledge and abilities that we can help them to uncover. In order to do this, we simply need to create an environment in which these inner resources can display themselves—a space of silence in which we can listen to and really meet the other person. This is a wonderful approach that helps us learn how to take care of the other, and in doing so to take care of ourselves; and taking care of ourselves teaches us how to better take care of the other. Slowly, through this dynamic relationship, we come to discover who we really are, because we are transformed by the richness of meeting and sharing with this other person. At the same time, we are perfectly at home in this process of helping others and helping them to grow. Because of these other people, we take on a renewed importance, and we are growing at the same time.

On the basis of this experience of care, the Tonglen Association has developed training modules to help us become what I would describe as better human beings. In our everyday lives, we are all going to come into contact with people who are suffering in different ways, and we can learn how to help them to live better and make their way through the chaos of life. In short, we learn how to care. After the training courses, some people decide to become volunteer caregiver-companions. We have also developed courses for health-care staff, and I will now describe one of these, which we named "Being, Presence, and Listening."

The course was developed with several important observations in mind. First, patients and people who are going through difficulties often complain more about a lack of listening from their caregivers than they do about their illness or other problems. Second, caregivers and health-care professionals dealing with suffering in their patients are frequently faced with an ever-increasing workload and cannot see how they can find the time to do everything. This is often a cause of stress and dissatisfaction, and burnout lurks just around the corner.

Meditation is a way of relating to our minds that enables us to face up to these challenges. We do not actually use the word *meditation* straightaway, as it can bring with it all sorts of ideas, concepts, and preconceptions, and these can get in the way. Instead, we talk about "taking a break," and every training session begins and ends with one of these "breaks." I'm going to suggest we take a break right now. . . .

Relaxation, Space, and Stability

You do not need to change your position. Simply become aware of your body as you sit on your chair. Just feel the contact of your backside on the seat, and the contact of your feet on the floor. That is all. It is not complicated or esoteric. Perhaps you are now becoming more aware of your body?

Now, become aware of the tension in your body. Did you know that the tension we carry in our bodies during the day, and even when we are asleep at night, is the equivalent of carrying a bag weighing between ten and twenty pounds around with us all the time. How does your jaw feel? And your shoulders? What about your belly? Gently relax as you breathe out.

The outbreath is a movement of relaxation. It is also a very important moment—for example, in martial arts—because it's the moment when you are stable and you can act. In the movement of relaxation, perhaps you can feel that something begins to unknot. Your feet are on the ground, your backside is firmly in contact with the seat, and you can feel the weight of your body. It is as if a space is being created inside us, where we can settle, quietly.

We can make use of this space to ask, *Why am I here?* Often, when we are busy doing things, we lose sight of our motivation and the intention we set out with. Just come back to that. *Why am I reading this book?* Or, *Why do I want to care for others?* In asking the question, something gets freed. Something opens up. It is as if your mind is able to change direction and say, *Ah, I lost my way.*

There really is nothing esoteric about all of this. It can take just a few seconds once we are used to it, and we do not have to do this for very long, but gradually we propose longer sessions so that people can fully experience it.

For more than ten years, we have been offering trainings on listening, being present, care, communication, and crisis management, and professionals have told us how beneficial they have found this approach to be, in both the short- and the long-term. Even in France—where the separation of church and state has been so strict, there has been so much confusion of spirituality with religion, and anything that goes off the beaten religious track is viewed almost as a cult or sect—it is encouraging to see that meditation is now receiving the recognition that it deserves.

We developed the "Being, Presence, and Listening" course for the ISFI Nord nursing school in Marseille.[1] We ran the course for the first time in 2007, with Geneviève Botti, and repeated it there and in other colleges over the following years. The course was for first-year students and consisted of seven three-hour modules, given over five months for two groups of twelve to fourteen students. Although it was a mandatory module, the students did not receive any credits toward their end-of-year exam, which was their main focus. Since offering the module was an innovative decision on the part of the management at the college, we also suggested carrying out an evaluation.

There is an unavoidable suffering in our lives, which is the suffering of our own limitations—of sickness, separation, change, and death. Often, however, the way we respond to the events that we encounter in our lives piles further suffering onto this suffering, and this can be prevented. When we realize the ways our mind does us a disservice rather than a service, we begin to see why it is important to learn to use it better, rather than let it use us. When we care for others, we learn how important it is to help them to realize this. It is vital, therefore, that this knowledge of the way our mind works be brought into the training that health-care professionals receive. Getting to know oneself and how to take care of oneself enables one to know and understand the other person, and therefore to care for this person better.

Recently, I was giving a two-hour presentation to about sixty fifth- and sixth-year medical students entitled "How to Be with People Who Are Suffering." I got them to see the point of taking a break, both for their own sakes and because this is the basis for a deeper and more generous quality of listening. After the two-hour presentation, several students got up and one of them started to speak, with a hint of anger in his voice. "It's scandalous that we only get taught this in the sixth year," he said. "We have accumulated huge amounts of knowledge and know-how, but *this* is absolutely fundamental. Why is it taught so late in the course, and so briefly?" The students were really moved, because the training they receive focuses only on knowledge and technical expertise, which can change as science progresses. They had never learned simply how to *be*, even though this is the basis for any encounter with a patient in order to establish a diagnosis. I took the student's anger to be a good sign.

To put it another way, by creating an environment that is conducive to listening, naturally we will understand better. Knowing oneself, understanding oneself, and taking care of oneself is truly the way to know, understand, and care for others. This is common sense, and this approach contributes to the right circumstances for healing. I am not going to go into detail about what we are healing, but there are different levels: healing the body, healing the heart, and healing the mind.

This brings to mind the story of Michèle, a well-known psychoanalyst in France. She was full of anger when she came to us, because she had just discovered that she had been lied to regarding her health status. Her test results had been altered, and in fact she had an advanced stage of cancer, which had metastasized in the liver. As a doctor, she knew exactly what that meant.

Michèle took part in one of our three- or four-day care seminars for people going through difficulties, in which we consider how to see things from a different perspective. At the end of her stay, she said, "I don't know if my cancer will be cured, and in fact I think I'm going to die, but already something has happened to me. I have discovered that silence leads to a quality of listening I had not imagined possible, and to a great deal of gentleness. It's like putting together all the pieces of a puzzle and seeing that it has a meaning. Everything seems much more simple."

Two days later, I received a call and was told, "Michèle has had a stroke and cannot speak anymore." For a psychoanalyst, talking is so important, and as I went to visit her I was thinking that it must be terribly difficult for her. When I went into her room I asked her, "How do you feel?" She looked at me with a big smile and gestured with her hand that everything was for the best. What had healed? Not her body, because she died the following day, but something inside had healed. She was deeply at peace.

In order to get to know ourselves better, and to know another person better, we ask ourselves, *Who are we?* The training course looks at this by using a number of contemplations about our perceptions, and how we deal with thoughts and emotions. By realizing how our minds work, and how our perceptions, emotions, and thoughts can take over and manipulate us, we see how this can lead to stress, suffering, and mistreatment. Quite naturally, we arrive at the conclusion that if we want to live better, we need to learn to see reality as it is, rather than as it appears or as we would like it to be; and we need to learn how to be, rather than simply loading ourselves up with knowledge. We can achieve this easily if we know how to calm and control our mind and make it more effective through meditation.

Meditation is extraordinary, because there is nothing more that we need to learn or do. In fact, it is a process of simplification. This is very good news when we are already so overwhelmed by all the other things that we are required to do or to know. Anyone who works in health care knows only too well how much heavier the load has become in recent times as a result of increasing administrative demands, reductions in staff, and so on. Perhaps, though, there is a way to do the same things with efficiency and kindness toward others, while at the same time avoiding exhaustion. We can learn to create space within ourselves from which we can open up and be one with the other person, listen, and let this person relax and find his or her place. We can nourish each other with this attitude, and we can experience the effects quite quickly.

I will now explain how we present some of the themes developed in the training. For the question *Who are we?* there is a lesson on perceptions called "Our Senses Are Tricking Us." We do not see reality as it is. We let ourselves be tricked into thinking that something is real, but in fact our perceptions cannot perceive it fully or are interpreting it. For example, we see only certain wavelengths that make up the color spectrum, and we only hear only a limited range of vibrations as sound, whereas some animals have a much wider range. So we are limited by our sense faculties.

We do not perceive the continuous changes that are happening in us. We are not exactly the same now as we were a few minutes ago. Did we perceive that change? We do not perceive everything that is moving around us. We do not feel the earth turning. It would make our lives more complicated, of course, if we were able to feel all these movements and changes, so we filter out this sort of information in order to function normally. But that also means we have to cut ourselves off from large amounts of information. So in a sense we have cut ourselves off from a part of what is real. There are many examples that prove that our brain repeatedly rebuilds the reality that it thinks most probable. We have a probabilist approach to what's around us, and so we do not see things as they really are.

The other theme that we develop in our training is that our senses build themselves through action, that is, we have to *do* in order to develop our senses. The experiments conducted by two psychologists, Richard Held and Alan Hein, in 1958 show this in a brilliantly simple way.[2] They reared a group of kittens in the dark, and allowed only some of them to move around freely. These kittens had small carts attached to them containing other kittens, who were not able to move about by themselves. After a few weeks, all the kittens were exposed to the light and allowed to move about freely. Only the kittens who had been allowed to move freely from the outset were now able to move about normally, as "sighted" kittens would. The ones who had been pulled around in the carts behaved as if they were blind, knocking into things and falling over. This experiment confirms that visual perception is developed on the basis of the visual guidance provided by activity. Similar results were obtained in other situations, even in studies conducted on single cells. So it seems that there is no external reality unless we are participating actively in the world.

We can develop this theme by reflecting on what happens whenever we do something for someone else: for our children, whom we try to protect from the pitfalls of life, or for our patients, who we feel are vulnerable.

The training session on perceptions reveals that we do not see reality as it is. Not only do we continuously filter the information we receive according to our habits and the urgency of other priorities at the time, but we also interpret things in different ways according to our history, our education, and our state of mind. In this way, each one of us arrives at our own vision of the world. With this in mind, we can better understand how difficult it is to communicate, and how important it is to develop our awareness and presence in order to improve our listening.

We dedicate another session to emotions. Looking at the difference between the limbic system and the cortical regions of the brain, we consider how our emotions often take us away from reason. That is why the neuroscientist Rita Levi-Montalcini, who was awarded the Nobel Prize for Physiology or Medicine in 1986, said that man is only a *Homo erectus* and not yet a *Homo sapiens*, because he is still enslaved by his irrational thoughts and emotions. In this context, we also consider the importance of being able to listen to patients' emotions, without fear but also without joining in—distinct but not distant.

In the third session we look at the idea that our thoughts, which we believe to be internal, actually interfere with our relationships with others. They are a constant background noise in our minds, disturbing our ability to think clearly and muddying or obstructing our communications. Our deepest values, the choices we make, our habits, and our experiences all impact on our actions, whether we are conscious of this or not. Even the way we access our memory depends upon our state of mind.

With this in mind, when we look at how to relate to others, we realize that the problem is not the information that we receive but how we interpret it. The same initially neutral stimulation, such as someone knocking at the door, will be interpreted differently according to what thought is in my mind at the time. The thought will produce an emotion, which will lead to a specific action. For example, if my neighbor has been having problems with some troublesome local youths, then I might think of them when I hear the knock, and I might be angry, tense, or anxious by the time I get to the door. On the other hand, if I am expecting a friend to call, it is likely I will open the door with a big smile on my face. And if I am afraid because I have heard about a wave of burglaries in the area, I might think someone is trying to break in.

We are constantly receiving large numbers of stimuli through our senses, and these cause thoughts to arise. As a result we are overwhelmed by all sorts of different emotions, which guide our actions without our even knowing it. Most of our actions, then, are automatic rather than deliberate. They are responses to stimuli, and most of the time they arise without our having any control over them. We think we are masters of our actions, thoughts, and choices, but how much freedom do we really have?

When it comes to the subject of ethics, we assume that reflection and discussion are all we need to get our ideas clear and decide upon the right action to take. However, there is a multitude of little moments in any given situation that influence its makeup and constantly make it change. As Francisco Varela outlines in his book, *Ethical Know-How,* we need to take each of these "microworlds" into account. They are the reality of our lives. Each of these moments generates countless different stimuli, leading to attitudes that are, as we have just seen, reactions rather than free actions. What is our attitude in each of these micromoments? Are we being ethical in this "immediate coping," as Varela describes it?

The communication that we establish with others, therefore, is always dependent on our state of mind, our interpretation, and our habitual tendencies. The way we behave cannot be separated from the way things and others appear to us. Once we see that we are enslaved and that we do not have much internal freedom, we can easily understand the value of learning to use our mind better. Armed with this knowledge, we see that there are countless moments when we do the opposite of what we would like to do, and when we are in fact mistreating others, either in our work or our daily life.

By teaching us how to be more present for ourselves and others, meditation enables us to observe our behavior, and to become more aware of it. This is not about judging oneself. It is about very gently bringing mindfulness, awareness, and space into whatever we are doing. Meditation leads us to adopt a radically different attitude toward ourselves and our environment. It is an extremely effective way to learn how to be more present for another person when faced with all the professional constraints that allow less and less time to devote to him or her. This attitude alone quite naturally creates a space where things can relax, unwind, and disarm themselves.

Space and silence are very powerful. There was a man called Diego who came to one of our care seminars. As someone with a Cartesian outlook on life, he only believed in what he had touched and understood. He gave us the following feedback about an exercise that involves silent face-to-face communication with another person:

> My Cartesian mind is troubled by it, even though I actually experienced it; and yet the feedback I have received proves that it works! For decades I have been used to taking decisions and giving direction. I was vaguely aware that people around me were suffering the consequences, but how do you summon up the will to change? You know better than I how deeply ingrained our behaviors are, but I wanted to tell you that I have begun to apply the moral pledges that I made. It's difficult, of course. The image that came to mind when I was doing the group exercise was that it felt exactly the same as when I was learning to parachute. When you are four thousand meters above the ground, staring out into empty space with the plane door open and a deafening noise in your ears, your head is saying "Do it!" and your body is screaming "No!" I'm probably the only one who really understands the internal struggle I went through in this situation. But in any case, everyone around me has been surprised to see the transformation!

That is indeed how we are, and I don't think there is anything wrong in acknowledging that we put up some resistance. There really is quite a struggle between our habits and our aspirations.

We evaluated our training program at the end of the first course of seven sessions. Each three-hour session comprised two parts, which started and finished with ten minutes of "break time," so students did seven forty-minute periods of meditation in total. That is not very much, and yet the evaluations we did one month and six months later showed that 70 percent of the students were completely satisfied, and 80 percent said they would recommend the course to a friend. At the outset they were all very preoccupied with their exams, and this compulsory course did not offer them any points toward it. Sixty-five percent said that they had tried out the meditation and that it had done them a lot of good. More than half had begun to take regular "breaks" in their lives.

We received some amazing feedback from the students about how the course had helped them. They said the course had given them well-being, new-found energy, better impulse control, greater understanding of their limits, reduced prejudice, and a more appropriate attitude. For one student, who had remained silent at the back of the class throughout all the lessons, it had been a lifeline. She was able to express that in those moments she could find a little tranquility in the midst of all the distress and violence she was facing in her life.

I will conclude with a story. About a year ago, the Tonglen Association was approached by the Palliative Care Unit in Montpellier, in Southern France. We were asked if one of our volunteers could come to visit the unit. They explained that they were facing an ethical issue with a patient who was demanding to go to Belgium for euthanasia, and his family did not know what to do. The man's name was Stéphane. He was about forty years old and was suffering from a neurodegenerative disease, which over the course of two years had left him able to move only his eyelids. He had been a sportsman, and loved life. His despair was understandable.

One of our volunteer caregivers went to see Stéphane. He told us that before going into Stéphane's room, he had invoked, from deep in his heart, what for him represented love and wisdom, so that he would be able to manifest the appropriate attitude. Conversation was difficult as Stéphane could not speak, and the only way to communicate was to show him letters of the alphabet, in order to construct words and sentences, letter by letter. When he entered the room, the suffering was palpable. "Stéphane confided that he was overcome with anger," the caregiver told us later.

> After an hour or more, I decided to explain to him about "taking a break," and then to practice for a few minutes with him, using the breath as a support. To my surprise, Stéphane was very open to trying this, and his face lit up. For a few moments, it seemed to give him a sort of inner space, which I had the feeling he had been searching for. When I asked him afterward to describe how he had felt, Stéphane's only words were "less pain." After two hours, I asked him if he wanted me to come back and see him again. Stéphane said to come back soon, in two days, and he welcomed the idea that two or three of us might spend time with him during the next visits. In his longing to escape his intolerable suffering, the fleeting experience of meditation had clearly interested him enough for him to specifically ask to continue with it when we came back.

From that moment on, Stéphane never again asked for euthanasia. Three volunteers took turns to guide him in regular meditation sessions at the hospital, and later at his home. In a short space of time, he was smiling again, he had a focus in life, and to the great surprise and satisfaction of the nursing staff, he lived for almost a year.

The physical and emotional change in Stéphane before and after the volunteers' visit was plain to see. Patients with this disease get a lot of mucus, and they are afraid of "drowning." Stéphane was very anxious about this, and he had to undergo suction every ten minutes. While he was meditating, however, the amount of mucus reduced, his breathing settled, and his face relaxed and shone.

The people who cared for Stéphane were really stunned to see the change in him. They invited us to the Palliative Care Unit to talk about our work, and in a sense we came to be looked upon as "specialists" in dealing with difficult situations.

Before he died, Stéphane agreed that we could share his story with others. He knew nothing about Buddhism and did not follow any kind of spiritual path, but he said that discovering meditation was the most beautiful present he had ever been given. It had given him the chance to find clarity and space within himself.

We have seen here that we can learn how to be more present for others, to adapt our attitude so we can be more "right" with them, while still staying in tune with ourselves and with the external constraints that are placed upon us. There really is a way to develop a more naturally ethical attitude—what Francisco Varela called "immediate coping." He wrote: "As a first approximation, let me say that a wise (or virtuous) person is one who knows what is good and spontaneously does it."[3]

As we conclude this chapter, perhaps we can take the time, as we do at the end of each care meeting or training day, to take one last break and think: even if I have been distracted, and even if I have retained just a fraction of what I have read here, is there something that has moved me, and that I would like to keep? Is there something that I would like to take with me and use to nourish myself? Let's simply take the time to do that now, silently wishing that we can put it into practice; and that the effort we have made may be a real contribution to the work of all those people throughout the world who are working to relieve suffering and to bring more peace, more humanity, and more love.

12

Being Present When We Care

Rosamund Oliver

What happens when you try to show a group of prison officers how to meditate? Rosamund Oliver describes her experiences of teaching "spiritual care" in the United Kingdom, and how meditation methods can help people working in demanding jobs cope with stress, compassion fatigue, and burnout.

It may be difficult to believe this now, but in the late 1970s and early 1980s "meditation" was still a dirty word in professional work. At best it was some benign, New Age hippie concept—weird but harmless—and at worst it was seen as the thin end of a wedge that would open the way for brainwashing and cult indoctrination.

Working in central London at this time, with access to yoga classes and meeting a growing number of people influenced by the spread of Buddhist thinking, I was part of a group of people who were discovering for themselves the power of meditation to bring more peace and relaxation into our very stressed and busy lives. I cannot easily describe what a radical and total shift this experience of discovery was for me, as it affected all levels of my being and the way I related to others. To integrate this shift with my life and work I had to spend several years studying first Zen and then Tibetan Buddhist methods of meditation before beginning to understand how they might be brought into the workplace.

Working at a meditation center in North London in 1984, I became part of a small group of people who began to share the meditation methods that we had learned with anyone who found their way to the weekly classes. This included a growing number of professionals working in a variety of occupations and institutions, such as social service, law, finance, teaching, hospitals, hospices, and prisons. Later, some of these people invited me back into their organizations to give talks or classes on meditation.

Meditation has a long history and comes from an oral tradition. It has been passed literally from mouth to ear, through lineages of teachers, for thousands of years, so you can say on one level that the instructions are a direct transmission. In 1978, I first learned the method of mindfulness meditation from Ajahn Sumedho, a teacher in the Thai Forest Tradition of Theravada Buddhism. Then I studied with a Zen teacher, focusing on practicing methods drawn from the *Sattipatthana Sutta*, which is the foundation of the Buddha's instructions for training in mindfulness. Since 1981 I have been studying in the Tibetan tradition with many teachers, including Sogyal Rinpoche, Chögyam Trungpa Rinpoche, Dilgo Khyentse Rinpoche, and His Holiness the Dalai Lama.

In more recent times, books have become key vehicles for the spread of this knowledge among a wider audience. When Sogyal Rinpoche's best-selling book, *The Tibetan Book of Living and Dying*, was published in 1992, there followed an increased demand for meditation classes in the centers that he had set up. In some places, people were queuing all the way down the road to get in, because they had read about the benefits of meditation in the book and now they wanted to learn how to do it. We can begin by reading about meditation, but somewhere along the line of learning how to do this we need to find someone who has practiced and understood meditation, and who can help us work with our understanding of what we have read. We need some form of instruction alongside our trying it out. It's a bit like learning to drive a car. It is much easier if we are shown how by someone who already drives.

Since the mid-1970s, many thousands of people have discovered meditation through the international network of centers, called Rigpa, that Sogyal Rinpoche has founded throughout the world (*rigpa* is a Tibetan word that means "the innermost nature of the mind"). Some might come to just one class, while others are still coming after twenty or thirty years. Either way, they get to meet meditation, and they can begin to understand the treasures of this extraordinary tradition.

Some people get hooked. The Zen teacher with whom I studied would often give us a warning before beginning a meditation talk. He would say, "Don't listen to this unless you are prepared to be hooked like a fish. If you are not ready to be caught, leave now." For many people, just hearing about meditation for the first time set them onto a completely new path of discovery that could be life-changing.

Because meditation has become much more widespread and more widely understood now, it is easy to forget the huge dedication that people made to find out more about these methods when they first made a connection with them, in some cases traveling for hours to attend classes. One man, a carpenter, made a round trip of four hundred miles to London and back every Thursday to learn how to meditate, in order to take the method back to a small group of people in Manchester, in the north of England.

Some people came because it was a cool thing to do, but they tended not to last for very long. More often, people came because they were stressed out or they had some distressing problems in their lives that they wanted to resolve. Some came after a huge crisis had rocked their lives. They did not come when they were right at the height of their crisis, for surviving often consumed all their energy and time. They would come afterward, as the crisis began to subside, because they wanted to find a way to help themselves to cope better with their lives or with such a problem in the future. An artist who came to a meditation class in London had been out one night and when he arrived back home he found there had been a fire and his house had completely burned down. All his artistic work had been destroyed, along with all his possessions. Understandably, he found the situation extremely difficult to cope with, and even more so when in the middle of all this his relationship ended as well. In other words, he lost everything. But he did not come to the meditation class right in the middle of that devastating situation. He came some months afterward, to learn the skills of meditation to help him cope as he put his life back together. These skills helped him move on from his huge loss and adapt to the complete change that had been forced upon him.

Some of the people who attended meditation classes in the early days worked in the health services, and they found that meditation brought great benefit to their lives. I remember a young doctor who came to one of the classes. At work, his colleagues were asking him, "What's going on? You seem to be so much more relaxed now." He said to me, "I can't tell them what I'm doing. They would think I was crazy if I said I was doing meditation." In those days, meditation and madness were not considered to be completely separate. If you were into meditation, it used to been seen as the beginning of a whole host of problems. It is wonderful nowadays that we can say we are doing meditation and people consider it to be something sane!

How did we begin to introduce these methods into the health-care system and other environments such as the prison system? First, the gradual acceptance of the idea of meditation was part of a seismic cultural shift that was happening in society at that time. Clearly there have been huge changes since World War II as we have made progress in dealing with poverty and illness, at least in the developed world. As these basic survival problems were improved and people started to live longer, the emphasis in affluent societies expanded to include other concerns, such as achieving greater well-being. In the United States, the United Kingdom, France, Germany, Australia, Switzerland, and other countries, interest grew in understanding how to increase contentment and happiness, both on an individual level and in social- and health-care provision. This focus went hand in hand with scientific research that proved the existence of links between increased well-being and practicing meditation.

Medical doctors, prison officers, nurses, social workers, and others across the world began to want to learn meditation methods, in order to improve their own well-being and their ability to cope with what were often stressful working conditions. Following the publication of *The Tibetan Book of Living and Dying*, the Spiritual Care Education Program was developed in several countries. This program was designed to bring the benefits of methods based on meditation and compassion into social- and health-care settings. We reflected on how we could take these methods into organizations and health services by encouraging and training professionals in how to use them at work. We wanted to show people working in such organizations, first, that they would benefit personally from having a simple daily meditation practice of their own and that this would also benefit those they looked after, and second, that if they learned some of the compassion practices that were outlined in the book, it would enhance the way they related to others, in either care or organizational work. We were also interested in showing how these methods could be used as antidotes to exhaustion and burnout.

It is important to point out that when we look after people on a deeper emotional or psychological level, we may still need to first address their physical misery and suffering. In *Uncompromising Truth for a Compromised World: Tibetan Buddhism and Today's World*, the Tibetan Buddhist teacher and scholar Professor Samdhong Rinpoche emphasizes this point with the following story:

> In the Pali Canon there is a story of a hungry man to whom Buddha would not give teaching. He said, "First you must feed him and he must be satisfied. Only after that will he be in a

> comfortable position, and then he will be able to listen to the teaching. So in the case of people who are consistently in poverty and misery we need to address the immediate miseries first. . . . Without fulfilling the basic needs of the body the mind is unable to get freedom from the painful demands of the body. This is a problem that underlies the nature of things, and we have to address it."[1]

In the environments in which medical workers, social workers, prison staff, and others are operating, very often they are confronting hunger, poverty, and suffering on different levels. Providing that level of care is very demanding on the people who work in these areas. According to the Health and Safety Executive, the national independent watchdog for work-related health, safety, and illness in the United Kingdom, the occupational fields that reported the highest rates of work-related stress in the three years from 2009 to 2011 were health, social work, education, and public administration. The occupations that reported the highest rates of work-related stress in those three years were health and social service managers, teachers, and professionals associated with providing social welfare.[2]

Many people in medical work and other related fields suffer from burnout and "compassion fatigue." Burnout is a state of ongoing physical, emotional, and mental exhaustion that does not seem to get better even after the sufferer has rested. It is strongly related to stress at work. Work, and even life in general, is experienced as overwhelming. It can lead to a state of depletion and fatigue that becomes defeatism, a feeling of hopelessness and helplessness, of being unable to find a way out of problems. This can be experienced so intensely that people are sometimes unable to continue to do their jobs, and they quit. Often unrecognized as it develops, burnout leaves people feeling negative about both themselves and their work, and they gradually lose touch with their own ability to feel compassion. This is sometimes called compassion fatigue, which has been described as untreated burnout. Often the most conscientious staff are the most vulnerable to burnout.

The people who came to our classes because they were performing stressful jobs found that they were not just learning skills that could be used to cope with stress at work, and that helped to prevent the buildup of burnout. They were also learning a whole raft of skills about a general way of being that was helping them to relate to many different situations and experiences in their lives. They realized that these methods might benefit others, too, and they wanted to pass them on to their work colleagues, as well as to their patients and clients.

When we first began to take these methods into hospitals and other organizations in order to show staff directly how to do this for themselves and their clients, we had to smuggle in the method of meditation. We could not even utter the word, because sometimes it created too much fear and suspicion. We had to call it something else, so we studied all kinds of different books to give us ideas for a terminology that would enable us to introduce these methods without using the word *meditation.* We settled on the term *stress management.*

Stress Management for Nurses

In 1987 I was invited to bring meditation methods into St. Joseph's, a large hospice in Hackney, East London. St. Joseph's was where Dame Cicely Saunders had first introduced her world-changing approach to pain management, which targeted all aspects of pain including social, emotional, and spiritual aspects of suffering. She was a pioneer in controlling the physical pain of dying people by using regular doses of analgesics such as morphine. At that time, St. Joseph's offered a course, recognized by the English National Board for Nursing, Midwifery and Health Visiting, on care for the dying patient. It was on this course, which we presented as "stress management," that I started to introduce the basic techniques of meditation—it would probably now be called mindfulness—to the nurses who came from all over the world to train at the hospice.

Two themes quickly emerged from the thirty or so nurses sitting quietly for five minutes, doing nothing except coming home to their own bodies and watching their breathing. First was a concern about how they spent time with patients. Some nurses recognized that they were so rushed in managing their workloads that they were not able to spend time just being with dying patients. They also felt they had to be perceived to be doing things, to be busy, and that simply sitting and being with a patient was not justifiable. One of the consequences of this style of working was that even when they wanted to pause and be present with a patient, the nurses found it very difficult to slow down and just do this. So we framed mindfulness meditation in the context of understanding Walter Cannon's fight-or-flight response; in the work of Hans Selye, the endocrinologist who first demonstrated the existence of stress; and boldly adapting Herbert Benson's method of "inducing the relaxation response." We then looked at practical ways to bring in this understanding for nurses. The intention was that nurses could learn new habits of mindfulness in work, and create ways to avoid overloading themselves, which would reduce the effects of stress. This would enable them to be more present with their patients and enhance the care they could give.

I shared a very simple method with the nurses called the Five-Minute Holiday. This method, developed by Sogyal Rinpoche, was a simple way people who were very busy could find time to sit quietly by themselves for five minutes a day and let their minds relax and ease as they focused their attention on one thing, such as their breathing. Having established this for themselves, they could then gradually extend the amount of time they spent sitting each day.

EXERCISE:

The Five-Minute Holiday

If you are new to meditation, or if you normally meditate with your eyes closed, you might like to try doing this with your eyes open. I would also encourage you to keep your back straight but not completely rigid, because that enables the energy in your body to flow better, and it helps your meditation if you can stay alert. If you feel your mind is quite busy, then you can direct your gaze slightly downward, and if you feel a bit sleepy, you can direct your gaze slightly upward.

We do this in three simple steps. Sogyal Rinpoche often says, "We are scattered everywhere and nobody's at home." So first, we *bring our mind home*. We simply allow all our scattered thoughts to come home, and let ourselves become more present. We are not thinking of the past, nor anticipating the future. As we do this, we can have a sense of being here, now, in our body, feeling our body on the seat. As we do this, we can feel the coziness and the deep sense of welcome in that. We do this for one minute.

Now for the second step: *release*. We release any holding or tension that we feel. We simply let go, in the same way we might let go of a clenched fist. As we breathe out, we let go of any tension at the same time; as we let go, we give ourself space. Just watching our breathing coming and going, we allow ourselves to experience a sense of spaciousness and openness. We can do this for two minutes.

Step three: *relax*. We let our mind settle naturally, welcoming whatever thoughts we find there. Being like a gracious host welcoming all the guests, giving each one perfect attention without spending too long talking to them, and then moving on to welcome the next one. Just easing into our natural self, our natural mind, the radiance of our fundamental nature, leaving our mind quietly, as much as we can, in a state of natural peace. We do this for another two minutes.

Now take a moment to check in with yourself. How does it feel to be like this? Does it feel natural? Is this a way you would want to continue to be in your life? A well-known Tibetan saying translates as, "Meditation is not, getting used to is." It is this spirit that we try to take into our practice, this sense of naturalness and of getting used to meditation.

As we finish our five-minute meditation, we try to take this feeling with us into our activity. Gradually, as we do this more in our life, we find we are doing things more naturally and a bit differently.

We can follow this method by bringing our attention to our breathing. However, not everyone is comfortable doing this, so instead we can use the method of focusing our attention on looking at an object, such as a vase of flowers, a pebble, or a candle—whatever works best for each person.

People found that sitting like this for just five minutes a day was a very powerful and simple way to help themselves slow down and become more centered and in touch with themselves. Afterward, as they went about their day, they found that this method enabled them to become more mindful, more aware of themselves, and, of course, more aware of how they were with others. The method also emphasized how to maintain this way of being more present in activity after the five minutes of sitting. Nurses discussed how they could integrate the flavor of this feeling into their work more. One method that was developed was to place a small colored paper dot on one's watch, so that every time a nurse looked to see the time, this marker was a reminder to pause and slow down, even for just a few seconds. Some members of staff thought that the practice of washing their hands, which was done frequently throughout the day, was a good reminder to slow down and reconnect with themselves. Another method was, when the phone rang, to pause for a second and breathe in and exhale before answering.

The second theme that emerged from the experience of sitting in meditation for five minutes was that nursing staff at the hospice were going through the experience of their patients' dying on a regular basis. Occasionally nurses would experience an overwhelming sense of loss when a patient died, and this unexpected response made them feel guilty because they felt it was unprofessional to feel such grief, so all they could do was bottle up their feelings. The holding down of these feelings became more apparent when these nurses spent even a short time meditating. So we looked at setting up simple support groups, which started with some quiet sitting, where nurses could talk privately about their experiences and receive shared support from their colleagues.

Meditation for Prison Staff

I also took these methods into other workplace settings. In 1992, a colleague who was a senior prison officer and I brought in these methods of mindfulness meditation as training for prison and probation officers and administrative staff at Pentonville Prison in North London, which currently has accommodation for more than 1,200 prisoners. Working in a prison is a high-stress job. Prison staff are known to have a high rate of heart disease, particularly those who have been in the service for a number of years, and studies have shown that they do not tend to live very long after they retire.[3] At Pentonville, the management had decided to tackle the problem of high stress levels and attrition rates among staff by creating a weekly opportunity for staff to spend an hour learning different de-stressing skills. This was known as "happy hour," which was not its official title, but the staff gave it that name. One of the options offered in this educational hour was learning physical and mental relaxation methods.

We still called the training "stress management." However, we began to use the word *meditation*, as we introduced a self-selected group of twenty staff members to different mindfulness meditation methods over a course of ten weekly sessions. We showed staff the method of the Five-Minute Holiday and specific ways of using breathing or looking at an object as a focus. Also, we daringly introduced what would now be called a body scan, and included one session where we used the method of meditating while listening to gentle music.[4]

Within each session, we provided a forum where staff members could discuss how they were using these methods and could get further guidance and encouragement where required. Many observed that they felt it was affecting them at quite a deep level, sometimes noticeable to others. One of the young officers reported, "The men on the landings said I am more relaxed than I was last month." They had asked him if he had been working out on exercise machines. Another older officer, who had suffered from severe tinnitus for several years, found that it improved considerably after a month of meditating daily. The program was judged to be very successful, and after the first ten weeks many of the prison officers and staff continued with a second and third course of instruction, learning to meditate under the guidance of the chief discipline officer at the prison.

This project lasted nearly two years. We found that when people working in the stressful work conditions of a prison were introduced to simple meditation methods, they became less stressed, more relaxed, and more able to relate to their colleagues and to the other people in their workplace, including the prisoners themselves. Not only did they find that they felt more relaxed and that their relationships with other people were easier; they also found that their ability to feel empathy and compassion for others increased, which seemed to be a natural component of meditation. When a gray-haired officer made a brief statement of fact, in one forum, about how meditating had finally enabled him to get in touch with the grief he felt over the loss of his wife, he was clearly surprised when others in the room encouraged him to talk more about his feelings. Their natural sympathy in the aftermath of meditating together seemed to enable him to make his disclosure.

Empathy and compassion can also be cultivated deliberately through meditation. One of the compassion methods we teach in the Spiritual Care Program is a short compassion contemplation, called *Seeing the other person as just another you.* It comes from a series of Buddhist practices designed to train the mind in developing compassion.

One of the most helpful ways to awaken our natural and inherent compassion is through this simple method of considering others as being the same as us. When we care for others we may feel that our compassion sometimes becomes blocked, and then we do not how to help the other person. Sometimes we can even forget that they are human, like us, and we look at them as just "numbers," or "patients." Instead of considering the other person in the light of all their history of pain and suffering, to which we may not know how to respond well, instead we can consider them simply as just another human being, just like us. If we can stop for even a minute and start considering the person in this way, it can really bring more human understanding, and our compassion often becomes unblocked.

We look at any other person with our mind's eye and see how he or she is just like us, with the same needs, the same fears, the same fundamental desire to be happy and to avoid suffering. When we take another step and put ourselves squarely in another person's shoes, we realize that just as we do not want suffering and long for happiness, so also that person wishes to avoid suffering and have happiness. Then we might feel more willing to be present with the person, to understand and accept him or her. As the Dalai Lama wrote, "After all, all human beings are the same—made of human flesh, bones and blood. We all want happiness and to avoid suffering. Further, we all have an equal right to be happy. It is important to realize our sameness as human beings."[5]

This meditation can open a door between us and any person with whom we have difficulty, and it can be especially helpful when we find it hard to get in touch with our compassion for someone, or even to imagine this person's suffering. It is also a good method to use when we are feeling burned out or overwhelmed by work, and even bogged down by the fact that there are so many people who need our care. If we can really consider each person that we are helping as unique, as just another one of us, and if we can remember just how much our care may mean to the person, it can inspire and transform us and help us to overcome exhaustion, because compassion is truly invigorating.

Before we begin this meditation, we choose one person to do this for. When we actually try to generate compassion for an individual, it can become challenging, so we can choose someone we would like to communicate with more but with whom we do not find it easy to talk. It could be a client, a patient, or a colleague at work. Perhaps we have a history with that person, or perhaps it is someone who pushes our buttons, or whom we do not know how to help, or someone who is very withdrawn or closed. When we are first training in this method, it is best not to pick someone who represents the most difficult challenge for us.

EXERCISE:

Seeing the Other Person as Just Another You

Start with a short period of sitting quietly and comfortably, alert but relaxed, just allowing yourself to become present. If it helps you to have your eyes closed, then you can do that.

First of all, reflect on the fact that we are all human. Each and every one of us is the same, in that we all want to be happy and we all want contentment, and we all wish to avoid pain and suffering.

Think of someone you wish to do this practice for, someone you know who is in difficulty in his or her life. You can imagine the person in front of you, just as you saw him or her recently. Try to feel that this person is present and with you now.

Consider how you would really like to communicate fully with this person. Ask yourself what gets in the way of communication. Is it a fear of being misunderstood? Or maybe you don't know what is getting in the way of communication. Notice whatever arises as you look at the person.

Now, instead of seeing this person in his or her usual role or way of being, consider him or her as just "another you." Consider that this person is the same as you.

This person has the same hopes and fears, the same deep desire for happiness, and for good circumstances in life. He or she also has the same deep fear of suffering, the same wish to be free of every kind of suffering and pain, with his or her own experience of fear, rejection, sadness, or anger. So in every way, you can consider that the person facing you is the same as you, just another you.

Now, you can open your heart, feeling compassion by wishing that this person could be free of his or her suffering. After staying with this feeling for a few moments, you can wish the person well and let the image of the person go, and just return to your sitting. And when you feel ready, just open your eyes and rest in any good feelings that you have.

This is a very simple compassion reflection that we can do quickly before we go to be with someone who is in pain or suffering. We can just flash onto it for a few seconds, remembering, *This person is the same as me. This person is just another me.*

If you wish to go further with this, for a few moments at the end of the meditation you can even put yourself in this person's shoes and imagine swapping places with her or him, becoming the person, seeing how the world is for this individual.[6]

I have tried to offer a glimpse of the richness of this ancient tradition that we are now inheriting. Teachers and experts steeped in the Buddhist tradition have brought this practical knowledge to the West over the past forty years or so. Gradually and patiently, they have shared these gems of meditation practice and the wisdom of compassion training, introducing these simple but subtle methods to us, in the hope that we would find ways to integrate them in our work and life here in the West. Particularly now, we can bring these methods imbued with wisdom and compassion into the world of health care and social care, to enhance the often excellent care provision that is already given to clients and patients. I have tried to show how these methods can provide care for the caregivers themselves and can be fully incorporated into self-care strategies as antidotes to burnout and stress. These methods can be used beneficially by those working in even the most difficult and stressful occupations such as prison work, and can improve the well-being of staff members, which will hopefully also have a beneficial effect on their relationships with their colleagues, families, and everyone they meet in the course of their work.

Finally, we are actively trying to spread this practical knowledge as widely as possible, and I think it is absolutely right to say that this is something we need to continue to commit to bringing to the West. For as Sogyal Rinpoche wrote in *The Tibetan Book of Living and Dying*:

> What is compassion? It is not simply a sense of sympathy or caring for the person suffering, not simply a warmth of heart toward the person before you, or a sharp clarity of recognition of their needs and pain, it is also a sustained and practical determination to do whatever is possible and necessary to help alleviate their suffering.[7]

Notes

INTRODUCTION

1. "They Thought Something Was Wrong with the Machine," *View: The Rigpa Journal*, no. 3 (August 2009): 42–47.
2. Antoine Lutz et al., "Long-Term Meditators Self-Induce High-Amplitude Gamma Synchrony during Mental Practice," *Proceedings of the National Academy of Science* 101, no. 46 (2004): 16369–73.
3. Joel Stein et al., "Just Say Om," *Time*, August 4, 2003, 48–56; James Shreeve, "Beyond the Brain," *National Geographic*, March 2005, 2–31.
4. The research mentioned in this list is presented in chapters 4 and 6 of this book.

CHAPTER 1

1. Shantideva, *Bodhicharyavatara: The Way of the Bodhisattva* (Boston: Shambhala, 1997), chapter 5, verses 2–3; see also verses 5–6.
2. *The Dhammapada: The Sayings of the Buddha*, translated by Thomas Byrom (Boston: Shambhala, 1993), chapter 1, verses 1–2.
3. William Shakespeare, *Hamlet*, act 2, scene 2, lines 256–57.
4. Shantideva, *Bodhicharyavatara*, chapter 1, verse 28.
5. John Milton, *Paradise Lost*, book 1, lines 254–55.
6. From "A Meeting of Minds: His Holiness the Dalai Lama and Professor Aaron T. Beck in Conversation," a video made at the International Congress of Cognitive Psychotherapy Convention 2005 (Göteborg, Sweden, June 13, 2005), www.youtube.com/watch?v=OyaD2kxEZcA.

7. Blaise Pascal, *Pensées*, no. 139.
8. The three methods—using an image, the sound of a mantra, and focusing on the breath—can also be combined into one, in what I have called the "Unifying Practice." See Sogyal Rinpoche, *The Tibetan Book of Living and Dying* (San Francisco: HarperSanFrancisco, 2002), 69–74.
9. Sogyal Rinpoche, *Tibetan Book of Living and Dying*, 73.
10. Longchenpa, "Self Liberation in the Nature of Mind" ("Semnyi Rangdrol").
11. Sogyal Rinpoche, *Tibetan Book of Living and Dying*, 76.

CHAPTER 3

1. See chapter 6.
2. Ibid.

CHAPTER 4

1. Clifford D. Saron and Richard J. Davidson, "The Brain and Emotions," in *Healing Emotions: Conversations with the Dalai Lama on Mindfulness, Emotions, and Health*, edited by Daniel Goleman (Boston: Shambhala, 1997), 67–88. To find out more about the Mind and Life Institute, visit www.mindandlife.org.
2. B. Alan Wallace describes shamatha meditation as "a path of attentional development that culminates in an attention that can be sustained for hours on end." B. Alan Wallace, *The Attention Revolution: Unlocking the Power of the Focused Mind* (Somerville: Wisdom Publications, 2006), xii.
3. EEG (electroencephalography) involves noninvasively recording and interpreting electrical activity originating from the brain using electrodes attached to the scalp surface. These minute oscillating "brain waves" can be used to estimate activation of different brain regions when the subject is resting or performing different perceptual, cognitive, or emotional tasks. Brain electrical activity shifts in a predictable pattern during the sleep-waking cycle. Repeated stimuli can be used to elicit

event-related brain potentials that reflect perceptual, cognitive, and motor processes related to task performance.

4. Zara Houshmand et al., "Training the Mind: First Steps in a Cross-Cultural Collaboration in Neuroscientific Research," in *Visions of Compassion: Western Scientists and Tibetan Buddhists Examine Human Nature*, edited by Richard J. Davidson and Anne Harrington (New York: Oxford University Press, 2001), 3–17.
5. The project was funded by Fetzer Institute grant 2191, and by gifts from the Hershey Family Foundation, the Tan Teo Foundation, the Yoga Research and Education Foundation, the Mental Insight Foundation, the Baumann Foundation, the Santa Barbara Institute for Consciousness Studies, Grant Couch and Louise Pearson, and Caroline Zecca-Ferris, as well as other individuals and anonymous donors. The Shamatha Project was additionally supported by an F. J. Varela research award from the Mind and Life Institute to Manish Saggar, a postdoctoral fellowship from the Social Sciences and Humanities Research Council of Canada to Baljinder K. Sahdra, and National Science Foundation predoctoral fellowships to Katherine A. MacLean and Anahita B. Hamidi. Sponsorship in the form of publicity for participant recruitment and discount services was provided by the Shambhala Mountain Center and an in-kind loan by the Mind and Life Institute.

   Project team since inception:

   Clifford Saron (principal investigator), University of California, Davis; and B. Alan Wallace (contemplative director), Santa Barbara Institute for Consciousness Studies.

   Additional investigators associated with the University of California, Davis: Karen Bales, Emilio Ferrer, G. Ron Mangun, Erika Rosenberg, and Philip Shaver.

   Scientific trainees at the University of California, Davis (with their current affiliations if not at UC Davis): Stephen Aichele; David Bridwell, Mind Research Network, Albuquerque,

N.M.; Hirokata Fukushima, Kansai University, Osaka, Japan; Anahita Hamidi; Tonya Jacobs; Brandon King; Shiri Lavy, Ariel University Center of Samaria; Katherine MacLean, Johns Hopkins University; Baljinder Sahdra, University of Western Sydney, Australia; Anthony Zanesco; Manish Saggar, Stanford University.

Consulting scientists and other investigators: Beth Adelson, Rutgers University; John J. B. Allen, University of Arizona; Ruth Baer, University of Kentucky; Elizabeth Blackburn, University of California, San Francisco; Jens Blechert, University of Salzburg, Austria; Richard Davidson, University of Wisconsin, Madison; Mingzhou Ding, University of Florida, Gainesville; Firdaus Dhabhar, Stanford University; Ezequiel di Paolo, Ikerbasque Basque Foundation for Science, San Sebastián, Spain; Paul Ekman, University of California, San Francisco; Elissa Epel, University of California, San Francisco; Barry Giesbrecht, University of California, Santa Barbara; Igor Grossman, University of Waterloo, Ontario, Canada; Paul Grossman, Basel University Hospital, Switzerland; Amishi Jha, University of Miami; Jue Lin, University of California, San Francisco; Margaret Kemeny, University of California, San Francisco; Antoine Lutz, Lyon Neuroscience Research Center, Lyon, France; Synthia Mellon, University of California, San Francisco; Gregory Miller, University of Delaware; Charles Raison, University of Arizona; Matthieu Ricard, Shechen Monastery, Nepal; Jonathan Schooler, University of California, Santa Barbara; Jonathan Smallwood, Max Planck Institute for Human Cognitive and Brain Sciences, Leipzig, Germany; Akaysha Tang, University of New Mexico; Ewa Wojciulik, Vanier College, Quebec; Owen Wolkowitz, University of California, San Francisco; Susan Bauer-Wu, University of Virginia.

6. The sand mandala is a Tibetan Buddhist practice in which special tools are used to painstakingly create a complex mandala from colored sand. Once completed, the sand mandala is carefully and ceremonially destroyed, to symbolize the transitory nature of material life.

7. These practices are described in detail in Wallace, *Attention Revolution,* and B. Alan Wallace, *The Four Immeasurables: Practices to Open the Heart* (Ithaca, N.Y.: Snow Lion Publications, 2010).
8. Attention tasks included the Stroop color and word test, the Eriksen flanker task, Covert Orienting Spatial Attention (Posner), continuous target detection line task, continuous target detection circle task, continuous response inhibition line task, the Operation Span task, and mind wandering tasks. Emotion tasks included emotion-primed lexical decision task, Microexpressions Test, emotion-modulated startle, Levenson and Ruef empathy task, emotional film cued-recall task, Implicit Attitude Test for fat-thin, and emotion-modulated attentional blink task.
9. Resiliency is described by the psychologists who created this questionnaire as being "as over-controlled as necessary and as under-controlled as possible." Jack Block and Adam M. Kremen, "IQ and Ego-resiliency: Conceptual and Empirical Connections and Separateness," *Journal of Personality and Social Psychology* 70, no. 2 (1996): 349–61.
10. Baljinder K. Sahdra et al., "Enhanced Response Inhibition during Intensive Meditation Predicts Improvements in Self-Reported Adaptive Socioemotional Functioning," *Emotion* 11, no. 2 (2011): 299–312.
11. Tonya L. Jacobs et al., "Self-Reported Mindfulness and Cortisol Dynamics during a Shamatha Meditation Retreat," *Health Psychology* (in press).
12. Elissa S. Epel et al., "The Rate of Leukocyte Telomere Shortening Predicts Mortality from Cardiovascular Disease in Elderly Men," *Aging* 1, no. 1 (2009): 81–88.
13. Elissa S. Epel et al., "Accelerated Telomere Shortening in Response to Life Stress," *Proceedings of the National Academy of Sciences of the United States of America* 101, no. 49 (2004): 17312–15.
14. Dean Ornish et al., "Increased Telomerase Activity and Comprehensive Lifestyle Changes: A Pilot Study," *Lancet Oncology* 9, no. 11 (2008): 1048–57.

15. Tonya L. Jacobs et al., "Intensive Meditation Training, Immune Cell Telomerase Activity, and Psychological Mediators," *Psychoneuroendocrinology* 36, no. 5 (2011): 664–81.
16. Elissa S. Epel et al., "Can Meditation Slow Rate of Cellular Aging? Cognitive Stress, Mindfulness, and Telomeres," *Annals of the New York Academy of Sciences* 1172 (2009): 34–53.
17. See Jon Kabat-Zinn and Mark Williams, eds., "Mindfulness: Diverse Perspectives on Its Meaning, Origins, and Multiple Applications at the Intersection of Science and Dharma," Special Issue, *Contemporary Buddhism: An Interdisciplinary Journal* 12, no. 1 (2011).
18. Ruth A. Baer et al., "Using Self-Report Assessment Methods to Explore Facets of Mindfulness," *Assessment* 13, no. 1 (2006): 27–45.
19. Carol D. Ryff, "Happiness Is Everything, or Is It? Explorations on the Meaning of Psychological Well-Being," *Journal of Personality and Social Psychology* 57, no. 6 (1989): 1069–81; Oliver P. John and Sanjay Srivastava, "The Big Five Trait Taxonomy: History, Measurement and Theoretical Perspectives," in *Handbook of Personality: Theory and Research*, 2nd ed., edited by Lawrence A. Pervin and Oliver P. John (New York: Guilford Press, 1999), 102–38.
20. Katherine A. MacLean et al., "Intensive Meditation Training Leads to Improvements in Perceptual Discrimination and Sustained Attention," *Psychological Science* 21, no. 6 (2010): 820–30. Katherine MacLean was a University of California, Davis, psychology graduate student when this study was initiated.
21. Katherine A. MacLean et al., "Effects of Intensive Meditation Training on Sustained Attention: Changes in Visual Event-related Potentials, Ongoing EEG and Behavioral Performance," program no. 873.1, *2009 Neuroscience Meeting Planner* (Chicago: Society for Neuroscience, 2009), available online.
22. Sahdra et al., "Enhanced Response Inhibition during Intensive Meditation."
23. Paul Ekman and Walter V. Friesen, "Measuring Facial Movement," *Environmental Psychology and Nonverbal Behavior* 1 (1976): 56–75.
24. Erika L. Rosenberg et al., "Meditation and the Plasticity of

Emotion: Facial Expression and the Unfolding of Emotional Responses to Suffering," in preparation.

25. My friend and colleague Paul Grossman, from University Hospital in Basel, Switzerland, and I thought up this name.
26. A wait list control group has been defined as follows: "In a study dealing with a therapy outcome, a wait list control group is a group that is assigned to a waiting list to receive an intervention after the active treatment group does. A wait list control group serves the purpose of providing an untreated comparison for the active treatment group, while at the same time allowing the wait-listed participants an opportunity to obtain the intervention at a later date" (http://depression.about.com/od/glossaryw/g/Wait-List-Control-Group.htm).
27. For details of the Inaugural Templeton Prize Research Grant supported by the John Templeton Foundation, see http://news.ucdavis.edu/search/news_detail.lasso?id=10420.

    For more information on the Shamatha Project: http://mindbrain.ucdavis.edu/labs/Saron/shamatha-project/.
28. I would like to thank Anahita Hamidi for her substantial, clarifying, and patient help in editing this chapter and Andy Fraser for further editing and guiding the process so smoothly.

CHAPTER 5

1. Discussed in more detail in chapter 6.
2. See chapter 4.
3. Tarthang Tulku, *Openness Mind: Self-Knowledge and Inner Peace through Meditation* (Cazadero, Calif.: Dharma Publishing, 1990), 51.

CHAPTER 6

1. Kimberly Goldapple et al., "Modulation of Cortical-Limbic Pathways in Major Depression," *Archives of General Psychiatry* 61, no. 1 (2004): 34–41.
2. Andrea Mechelli et al., "Structural Plasticity in the Bilingual Brain: Proficiency in a Second Language and Age at Acquisition Affect Grey-Matter Density," *Nature* 431 (2004): 757;

Christian Gaser and Gottfried Schlaug, "Brain Structures Differ between Musicians and Non-Musicians," *Journal of Neuroscience* 23, no. 27 (2003): 9240–45.

3. Bogdan Draganski et al., "Changes in Grey Matter Induced by Training," *Nature* 427 (January 2004): 311–12.
4. Stefan J. Borgwardt et al., "Regional Gray Matter Volume in Monozygotic Twins Concordant and Discordant for Schizophrenia," *Biological Psychiatry* 67, no. 10 (2009): 956–64.
5. Britta K. Hölzel et al., "Investigation of Mindfulness Meditation Practitioners with Voxel-Based Morphometry," *Social Cognitive and Affective Neuroscience* 3, no. 1 (2008): 55–61.
6. Britta K. Hölzel et al., "Mindfulness Practice Leads to Increases in Regional Brain Gray Matter Density," *Psychiatry Research: Neuroimaging* 191, no. 1 (2011): 36–43.
7. Rupshi Mitra et al., "Stress Duration Modulates the Spatiotemporal Patterns of Spine Formation in the Basolateral Amygdala," *Proceedings of the National Academy of Sciences of the United States of America* 102, no. 26 (2005): 9371–76.
8. Ajai Vyas et al., "Recovery after Chronic Stress Fails to Reverse Amygdaloid Neuronal Hypertrophy and Enhanced Anxiety-like Behavior," *Neuroscience* 128, no. 4 (2004): 667–73.

CHAPTER 7

1. In the present context, to recognize the universal character and applicability of the dharma, I am using the term with a lowercase *d*, except in those very specific circumstances where it signifies the traditional Buddhist teachings within an explicitly Buddhist context. See Jon Kabat-Zinn, "Some Reflections on the Origins of MBSR, Skillful Means, and the Trouble with Maps," in Mark Williams and Jon Kabat-Zinn, *Mindfulness: Diverse Perspectives on Its Meaning, Origins, and Applications* (London: Routledge, 2013), 281–306, first published as a Special Issue on Mindfulness in *Contemporary Buddhism* 12, no. 1 (2011).
2. See Jon Kabat-Zinn, "Orthogonal Reality—Rotating in Consciousness," in Jon Kabat-Zinn, *Coming to Our Senses: Healing*

Ourselves and the World through Mindfulness (New York: Hyperion, 2005), 347–52.

3. Francisco Varela (1946–2001) was cofounder of the Mind and Life Institute and a polymath of a thinker, philosopher, scientist, and Dharma practitioner. See Francisco Varela, Evan Thompson, and Eleanor Roach, *The Embodied Mind* (Cambridge, Mass.: MIT Press, 1992; 2nd edition, 2013).
4. Descartes was the father of the philosophical view that reality was split into the *res cogitans*, often translated as "thought substance," the domain of the immaterial, of mind or soul, of consciousness, and the *res extensa*, often translated as "extended substance," or material substance, the domain of the body and the world. This inaugurated a split between the domain of mind and the domain of body, a fundamentally dualistic, if totally understandable view that influenced Western scientific thought for centuries. It is only now that this view is succumbing to new understandings in biology that there is no fundamental separation between mind and body, although the split is maintained in our very use of language, and such words as *mind* and *body*, which already make them seem fundamentally separate. How consciousness arises from the material brain is as much a mystery as it ever was.
5. The first Noble Truth of the Buddha is that there is suffering. Here is the Buddha's classical definition of *dukkha*: "Now this, monks, is the Noble Truth of dukkha: Birth is dukkha, aging is dukkha, death is dukkha; sorrow, lamentation, pain, grief, and despair are dukkha; association with the unbeloved is dukkha; separation from the loved is dukkha; not getting what is wanted is dukkha. In short, the five clinging-aggregates are dukkha" (www.accesstoinsight.org/ptf/dhamma/sacca/sacca1/index.html).
6. Right or wise view, intention, speech, action, livelihood, effort, mindfulness, and concentration.
7. Jon Kabat-Zinn, *Full Catastrophe Living: Using the Wisdom of Your Body and Mind to Face Stress, Pain and Illness* (New York: Dell, 1990), 163.

8. Jon Kabat-Zinn, *Mindfulness for Beginners* (Boulder: Sounds True, 2011), 18; Kabat-Zinn, *Full Catastrophe Living*, 96–97.
9. Georges Dreyfus, "Is Mindfulness Present-centered and Non-judgmental? A Discussion of the Cognitive Dimensions of Mindfulness," in Williams and Kabat-Zinn, *Mindfulness*, 41–54.
10. John Dunne, "Toward an Understanding of Non-dual Mindfulness," in Williams and Kabat-Zinn, *Mindfulness*, 71–88.
11. Jon Kabat-Zinn and Richard J. Davidson, *The Mind's Own Physician: A Scientific Dialogue with the Dalai Lama on the Healing Power of Meditation* (Oakland, Calif.: New Harbinger, 2011), 56–57.
12. John D. Teasdale and Michael Chaskalson, "How Does Mindfulness Transform Suffering? I: The Nature and Origins of *Dukkha*," in Williams and Kabat-Zinn, *Mindfulness*, 89–102; John D. Teasdale and Michael Chaskalson, "How Does Mindfulness Transform Suffering? II: The Transformation of *Dukkha*," in Williams and Kabat-Zinn, *Mindfulness*, 103–24.
13. Jon Kabat-Zinn, foreword to Donald McCown, Diane Reibel, and Marc S. Micozzi, *Teaching Mindfulness* (New York: Springer, 2010), xix.
14. See Daniel Goleman, ed., *Healing Emotions: Conversations with the Dalai Lama on Mindfulness, Emotions and Health* (Boston: Shambhala, 2003), 113–44.
15. Various agencies put world population in 2012 at about 7 billion. In 1990 the population figure was approximately 5.5 billion.
16. Goleman, *Healing Emotions*, 189–200.
17. Mark Allen et al., "Participants' Experiences of Mindfulness-Based Cognitive Therapy: 'It Changed Me in Just about Every Way Possible,'" *Behavioural and Cognitive Psychology* 37 (2009): 413–30.
18. See notes 9 and 10, for example.
19. Jon Kabat-Zinn, "Two Ways to Think about Meditation," in *Coming to Our Senses*, 64–68.
20. Bhikkhu Bodhi, "What Does Mindfulness Really Mean? A Canonical Perspective," in Williams and Kabat-Zinn, *Mindfulness*, 19–39.
21. Jon Kabat-Zinn et al., "Influence of a Mindfulness-Based Stress

Reduction Intervention on Rates of Skin Clearing in Patients with Moderate to Severe Psoriasis Undergoing Phototherapy (UVB) and Photochemotherapy (PUVA)," *Psychosomatic Medicine* 60, no. 5 (1998): 625–32.

22. Britta K. Hölzel et al., "Mindfulness Practice Leads to Increases in Regional Brain Gray Matter Density," *Psychiatry Research* 191, no. 1 (2011): 36–43; Britta K. Hölzel et al., "Stress Reduction Correlates with Structural Changes in the Amygdala," *Social Cognitive Affective Neuroscience* 5, no. 1 (2010): 11–17.
23. Melissa A. Rosenkranz et al., "A Comparison of Mindfulness-based Stress Reduction and an Active Control in Modulation of Neurogenic Inflammation," *Brain Behavior and Immunity* 27 (2013): 174–84.
24. Jon Kabat-Zinn, "Participatory Medicine," *Journal of the European Academy of Dermatology and Venereology* 14 (2000): 239–40.
25. See "Healing the Body Politic," in Kabat-Zinn, *Coming to Our Senses*, 499–580.
26. Further studies and resources on mindfulness:

Jon Kabat-Zinn, "An Outpatient Program in Behavioral Medicine for Chronic Pain Patients Based on the Practice of Mindfulness Meditation: Theoretical Considerations and Preliminary Results," *General Hospital Psychiatry* 4, no. 1 (1982): 33–47.

Jon Kabat-Zinn, Leslie Lipworth, and Robert Burney, "The Clinical Use of Mindfulness Meditation for the Self-Regulation of Chronic Pain," *Journal of Behavioral Medicine* 8, no. 2 (1985): 163–90.

Jon Kabat-Zinn et al., "Four Year Follow-Up of a Meditation-Based Program for the Self-Regulation of Chronic Pain: Treatment Outcomes and Compliance," *Clinical Journal of Pain* 2, no. 3 (1986): 159–73.

Jon Kabat-Zinn and Ann Chapman-Waldrop, "Compliance with an Outpatient Stress Reduction Program: Rates and Predictors of Completion," *Journal of Behavioral Medicine* 11, no. 4 (1988): 333–52.

Richard J. Davidson et al., "Alterations in Brain and Immune

Function Produced by Mindfulness Meditation," *Psychosomatic Medicine* 65, no. 4 (2003): 564–70.

Jon Kabat-Zinn, "Mindfulness-Based Interventions in Context: Past, Present, and Future," *Clinical Psychology: Science and Practice* 10, no. 2 (2003): 144–56.

David S. Ludwig and Jon Kabat-Zinn, "Mindfulness in Medicine," *Journal of the American Medical Association* 300, no. 11 (2008): 1350–52.

CHAPTER 9

1. Aaron T. Beck et al., *Cognitive Therapy of Depression* (New York: Guilford Press, 1979); Christine Favre and Lucio Bizzini, "Some Contributions of Piaget's Genetic Epistemology and Psychology to Cognitive Therapy," *Clinical Psychology and Psychotherapy* 2, no. 1 (1995), 15–23.
2. Michael E. Addis and Christopher R. Martell, *Overcoming Depression One Step at a Time: The New Behavioral Activation Approach to Getting Your Life Back* (Oakland, Calif.: New Harbinger Publications, 2004).
3. Jeremy D. Safran and Zindel V. Segal, *Interpersonal Processes in Cognitive Therapy* (New York: Basis Books, 1990), 117.
4. Zindel V. Segal, John D. Teasdale, and J. Mark G. Williams, *Mindfulness-Based Cognitive Therapy for Depression: A New Approach to Preventing Relapse* (New York: Guilford Press, 2002); Jeremy D. Safran, "Psychoanalysis and Buddhism as Cultural Institutions," in *Psychoanalysis and Buddhism: An Unfolding Dialogue*, edited by Jeremy D. Safran (Somerville: Wisdom Publications, 2003).
5. Jean Piaget and Bärbel Inhelder, *The Child's Conception of Space* (Paris: PUF, 1948).
6. For a fuller description of the "raisin exercise," see p. 133.
7. Lucio Bizzini, Véra Bizzini, and Christine Favre, *Comment soigner la dépression gériatrique: Le manuel de traitement de groupe CTDS (Cognitive Therapy with Decentering Strategies)* (Geneva: Trajets, 1999), 66.

8. Segal et al., *Mindfulness-Based Cognitive Therapy for Depression*, 109–10.
9. Lucio Bizzini et al., "Mindfulness et dépression," *Santé mentale*, no. 147 (2010): 69–72; Guido Bondolfi et al., "Depression Relapse Prophylaxis with Mindfulness-Based Cognitive Therapy: Replication and Extension in the Swiss Health Care System," *Journal of Affective Disorders* 122, no. 3 (2010): 224–31.
10. Pierre Philippot and Zindel V. Segal, "Mindfulness-Based Psychological Interventions: Developing Emotional Awareness for Better Being," *Journal of Consciousness Studies* 16, no. 10–12 (2009): 285–306.
11. Segal et al., *Mindfulness-Based Cognitive Therapy for Depression*, 206.
12. Rumi, "The Guest House," from *Selected Poems: The Essential Rumi*, translated by Coleman Barks (New York: Penguin Classics, 2004), 109.
13. Segal et al., *Mindfulness-Based Cognitive Therapy for Depression*, 202.
14. See James Carmody and Ruth A. Baer, "Relationships between Mindfulness Practice and Levels of Mindfulness, Medical and Psychological Symptoms and Well-being in a Mindfulness-Based Stress Reduction Program," *Journal of Behavioral Medicine* 31, no. 1 (2008): 23–33; Filip Raes et al., "Mindfulness and Reduced Cognitive Reactivity to Sad Mood: Evidence from a Correlational Study and a Non-Randomized Waiting List Controlled Study," *Behaviour Research and Therapy* 47, no. 7 (2009): 623–27.
15. Emily L. B. Lykins and Ruth A. Baer, "Psychological Functioning in a Sample of Long-Term Practitioners of Mindfulness Meditation," *Journal of Cognitive Psychotherapy* 23, no. 3 (2009): 226–41.
16. James Carmody, "Evolving Conceptions of Mindfulness in Clinical Settings," *Journal of Cognitive Psychotherapy* 23, no. 3 (2009): 270–80.
17. For further reading:

    Jon Kabat-Zinn, *Full Catastrophe Living: Using the Wisdom of Your Body and Mind to Face Stress, Pain and Illness* (New York: Dell, 1990).

Jon Kabat-Zinn, *Wherever You Go, There You Are: Mindfulness Meditation in Everyday Life* (New York: Hyperion, 1994).

J. Mark G. Williams et al., *The Mindful Way through Depression: Freeing Yourself from Chronic Unhappiness* (New York: Guilford, 2007).

CHAPTER 10

1. Sogyal Rinpoche, *The Tibetan Book of Living and Dying* (HarperSanFrancisco, 2002), 69–74.
2. Stan Tomamdl, *Coma Work and Palliative Care* (N.p.: Interactive Media, 1991), available from the author; see www.comacommunication.com for contact information.
3. Caroline Garland, *Understanding Trauma: A Psychoanalytic Approach* (London: Karnac Books, 2004), 10.
4. Gaston Bachelard, *The Poetics of Space* (Boston: Beacon Press, 1994), xix.
5. Rainer Maria Rilke, *Letters to a Young Poet*, trans. M. D. Herter Norton (New York: W. W. Norton and Co., 2004), 52.
6. Thomas F. Walshe, *Favourite Poems We Learned in School* (Cork, Ireland: Mercier Press Ltd., 1993), 44.
7. Irvin D. Yalom and Carlos Greaves, "Group Therapy with the Terminally Ill," *American Journal of Psychiatry* 134, no. 4 (1977): 396–400.
8. Scott R. Bishop et al., "Mindfulness: A Proposed Operational Definition," *Clinical Psychology: Science and Practice* 11, no. 3 (2004): 230–41.
9. For further reading:

    Ruth A. Baer, "Mindfulness Training as a Clinical Intervention: A Conceptual and Empirical Review," *Clinical Psychology: Science and Practice* 10, no. 2 (2003): 125–43.

    Trish Bartley, *Mindfulness-Based Cognitive Therapy for Cancer* (Chichester, UK: Wiley-Blackwell, 2011).

    Richard J. Davidson et al., "Alterations in Brain and Immune Function Produced by Mindfulness Meditation," *Psychosomatic Medicine* 65, no. 4 (2003): 564–70.

Mircea Eliade, *The Myth of the Eternal Return: Cosmos and History*, translated by Willard R. Trask (Princeton: Princeton University Press, 1971).

Viktor E. Frankl, *Man's Search for Meaning* (London: Hodder & Stoughton, 2006).

Paul Grossman et al., "Mindfulness-Based Stress Reduction and Health Benefits: A Meta-Analysis," *Journal of Psychosomatic Research* 57, no. 1 (2004): 35–43.

Jon Kabat-Zinn, *Full Catastrophe Living: Using the Wisdom of Your Body and Mind to Face Stress, Pain and Illness* (New York: Dell, 1990).

Jon Kabat-Zinn, *Wherever You Go, There You Are: Mindfulness Meditation in Everyday Life* (New York: Hyperion, 1994).

Robert Kegan, *The Evolving Self* (Cambridge, Mass.: Harvard University Press, 1982).

Saki F. Santorelli, *Heal Thy Self* (New York: Bell Tower, 1999).

J. Mark G. Williams et al., *The Mindful Way through Depression: Freeing Yourself from Chronic Unhappiness* (New York: Guilford, 2007).

CHAPTER 11

1. IFSI (Institut de Formation en Soins Infirmiers) is a French association for the training of nurses. The training experience at the IFSI Nord nursing school in Marseille was described in Geneviève Botti et al., "Prévention du stress, une experience en formation infirmiere (Stress Prevention: An Experience in Nursing Education)," *Soins—La Revue de Reference Infirmiere*, no. 736 (June 2009): 24–27.
2. Richard Held and Alan Hein, "Movement-Produced Stimulation in the Development of Visually Guided Behavior," *Journal of Comparative and Physiological Psychology* 56, no. 5 (1963): 872–76.
3. Francisco Varela, *Ethical Know-How: Action, Wisdom, and Cognition* (Stanford University Press, 1999), 4.

CHAPTER 12

1. Samdhong Rinpoche, *Uncompromising Truth for a Compromised World: Tibetan Buddhism and Today's World* (Bloomington: World Wisdom, 2006), 200.
2. Health and Safety Executive Web site: www.hse.gov.uk/statistics/causdis/stress/index.htm.
3. According to the Prison Officers Association, in the U.K., the average life expectancy for its members after retirement is eighteen months to two years. These figures are supported by an investigation by the U.S. National Institute of Corrections, which found that after twenty years of service, the life expectancy of the average correctional officer was fifty-eight years of age (see Tony Thompson, "Poor Food and Stress 'Responsible for Rising Number of Deaths in UK Prisons,'" *The Observer,* August 8, 2010).
4. This particular method of using music as a focus was shown to us by Ato Rinpoche, a Tibetan meditation teacher living in Cambridge, who at that time taught monthly meditation days in our London center.
5. H.H. Dalai Lama, *A Policy of Kindness* (Ithaca, N.Y.: Snow Lion Publications, 1990), 48.
6. Meditation based on the practice described by Sogyal Rinpoche in *The Tibetan Book of Living and Dying* (HarperSanFrancisco, 2002), 200.
7. Ibid., 191.

About the Contributors

URSULA BATES is a clinical psychologist and group analyst with an interest in the field of psycho-oncology and staff development. She is the director of psychosocial and bereavement services at Blackrock Hospice in Dublin, Ireland, and provides a clinical service to the palliative-care patients at St. Vincent's University Hospital, Dublin. In 2003 she introduced mindfulness-based approaches for oncology and palliative patients and bereaved caregivers in a publicly funded health service in Ireland, at St. Vincent's and Blackrock Hospice.

LUCIO BIZZINI is a psychologist, psychotherapist, and founding member of the Swiss Association of Cognitive Psychotherapy. He practices in the Department of Psychiatry of the University Hospitals of Geneva, Switzerland, where he works in the Depression Treatment Program. He has been treating patients suffering from depression for more than twenty years and was among the first Mindfulness-Based Cognitive Therapy teachers trained by the pioneers of this approach.

Dr. Bizzini has been organizing MBCT groups since 2000 for patients suffering from depression. He offers numerous courses, workshops, and retreats in collaboration with the originators of this approach (Zindel Segal and Mark Williams) and with colleagues in Switzerland, France, Belgium, and Italy. He is an honorary member of the Association for the Development of Mindfulness.

CATHY BLANC is a practicing doctor, homeopath, and acupuncturist. In 1994 she founded the Tonglen Association, which translates universal human and spiritual values into secular care for those who are terminally ill or are experiencing difficulties. Besides its work with individuals, the Tonglen Association also collaborates closely with several hospital units in France to develop values such as compassion, presence, and deep listening within training programs for health-care professionals.

In addition to serving as president of the Tonglen Association, Dr. Blanc is a senior instructor, French national coordinator, and international training manager in Rigpa's Spiritual Care Education Program and gives many talks in this capacity. She is also invited by other organizations to lead seminars on care, as well as trainings in crisis management. She gives workshops, conferences, and professional seminars for health-care professionals and social workers in Europe on a regular basis. She has been practicing meditation in the Christian tradition since the late 1970s, and Tibetan Buddhist meditation since 1989.

DANIEL GOLEMAN is an internationally known psychologist who lectures frequently to professional groups and business audiences and on college campuses. An award-winning science journalist, he reported on the brain and behavioral sciences for the *New York Times* for many years. His book *Emotional Intelligence* has been a best seller in many countries. He has also written books on self-deception, creativity, transparency, meditation, social and emotional learning, ecoliteracy, and the ecological crisis.

Goleman is a cofounder of the Collaborative for Academic, Social, and Emotional Learning, now at the University of Illinois at Chicago. CASEL's mission is bringing evidence-based programs in emotional literacy to schools worldwide. He currently codirects the Consortium for Research on Emotional Intelligence in Organizations at Rutgers University. The consortium fosters research partnerships between academic scholars and practitioners on the role emotional intelligence plays in excellence.

He is a board member of the Mind and Life Institute, which fosters dialogues and research collaborations among contemplative practitioners and scientists. He has organized a series of intensive conversations between H.H. the Dalai Lama and scientists, which resulted in the books *Healthy Emotions* and *Destructive Emotions.* He is currently editing a book that emerged from the Mind and Life Institute dialogue in 2011 on ecology, interdependence, and ethics.

Jon Kabat-Zinn is a scientist, writer, and meditation teacher engaged in bringing mindfulness into the mainstream of medicine and society. He gives public talks and workshops throughout the world on mindfulness and its applications. He is professor emeritus of medicine at the University of Massachusetts Medical School, in Worcester, Massachusetts, where he was the founding executive director of the Center for Mindfulness in Medicine, Health Care, and Society and founder of its world-renowned Stress Reduction Clinic. He is also a board member of the Mind and Life Institute.

He is the author of numerous books, including *Full Catastrophe Living: Using the Wisdom of Your Body and Mind to Face Stress, Pain and Illness* and *Wherever You Go, There You Are: Mindfulness Meditation in Everyday Life.* He is the coauthor, with Richard Davidson, of *The Mind's Own Physician: A Scientific Dialogue with the Dalai Lama on the Healing Power of Meditation,* and coauthor, with his wife, Myla, of *Everyday Blessings: The Inner Work of Mindful Parenting.*

Kabat-Zinn's work has contributed to a growing movement of mindfulness in major fields and institutions in our society, such as the law, professional sports, medicine, health care and hospitals, schools, corporations, and prisons.

Sara W. Lazar is a neuroscientist in the psychiatry department at Massachusetts General Hospital and an instructor in psychology at Harvard Medical School. Her research focuses on studying the neural mechanisms underlying yoga and meditation, both in clinical settings and in healthy individuals, with emphasis on promoting and preserving their health and well-being. One main focus of her work is determining how yoga and meditation influence brain structure, and how these changes influence behavior. She has been practicing yoga and mindfulness meditation since 1994, and is a board member of the Institute for Meditation and Psychotherapy.

Edel Maex is a psychiatrist at the ZNA St. Elisabeth Hospital in Antwerp, Belgium. He is a longtime practitioner of Zen Buddhism and a student of Frank De Waele Sensei, in the White Plum Tradition. He has become well known as a pioneer in mindfulness training in a medical setting and is the author of a stress-reduction manual published in Dutch, *Relieving Stress through Mindfulness: An Eight-Week Training Programme (Mindfulness, in de maalstroom van je leven),* which has been translated into French and German. He is secretary general of the Buddhist Union of Belgium.

Rosamund Oliver is a United Kingdom Council for Psychotherapy (UKCP) registered psychotherapist and supervisor and holds a European Certificate of Psychotherapy (ECP). She has worked with elderly bereaved patients in a large London teaching hospital, taught nurses at St. Joseph's Hospice, and jointly created and led a prison meditation project.

As an international trainer for Rigpa's Spiritual Care Program, she gives seminars to professionals in many countries. She has led Buddhist psychotherapy seminars in South Africa. She has done extensive training in meditation and Buddhism, including attending a three-year retreat. She has been a student of the Tibetan Buddhist teacher Sogyal Rinpoche since 1981 and is an international senior instructor for Rigpa. She has also been given the Freedom of the City of London in recognition of her work there.

Jetsün Khandro Rinpoche is the eldest daughter of the late Mindrolling Trichen, who was the holder of the Mindrolling lineage, one of the six main lineages of the Nyingma school of Tibetan Buddhism. She has been teaching extensively from both the Kagyu and Nyingma traditions in North America, Europe, and Asia since 1992.

Khandro Rinpoche has established and heads the Samten Tse

Retreat Center in Mussoorie, India, which provides a place of study and retreat for monastics and lay practitioners from the East and West. She is also the founder of the Lotus Garden Retreat Center in rural Stanley, Virginia, and is actively involved with the administration of Mindrolling Monastery in Dehra Dun, India. She is the author of *This Precious Life: Tibetan Buddhist Teachings on the Path to Enlightenment.*

Khandro Rinpoche also heads a variety of charitable projects, including support for leprosy patients, home and health care for the elderly, construction of hospitals and schools, and sponsoring students and monastics.

SOGYAL RINPOCHE is one of the best-known Buddhist teachers of our time. Born and raised in Tibet, he studied with many of the greatest masters of the twentieth century, including Jamyang Khyentse Chökyi Lodrö, Dudjom Rinpoche, and Dilgo Khyentse Rinpoche. In 1971 Sogyal Rinpoche went to England, where he studied comparative religion at Cambridge University. He has spent almost forty years traveling to many countries around the world, sharing the wisdom of the Buddha's teachings and introducing meditation to thousands of people.

Sogyal Rinpoche is the founder and spiritual director of Rigpa, an international network of more than 130 Buddhist centers and groups in forty-one countries around the world. His groundbreaking book, *The Tibetan Book of Living and Dying*, has been acclaimed as a spiritual classic. Three million copies have been printed in thirty-four languages, and the book is available in eighty countries.

ERIKA ROSENBERG is an emotions researcher, health psychologist, educator about emotional life, and an expert in facial expression measurement using the Facial Action Coding System. In her research on emotion she has examined how our feelings are revealed in our facial expressions, how social factors influence emotional signals, and how anger affects cardiovascular health.

Rosenberg is a researcher at the Center for Mind and Brain at the University of California, Davis, and a senior investigator on the Shamatha Project, a multidisciplinary study of how intensive meditation affects cognition, emotion, and neurophysiology. She is coauthor and senior teacher of the Compassion Cultivation Training course developed at Stanford University. She has been practicing meditation for more than twenty years and serves on the faculty of the Nyingma Institute of Tibetan Studies in Berkeley, where she teaches meditation courses and holds workshops in the development of mindfulness and compassion, and in working with emotions in daily life.

Frédéric Rosenfeld is a physician and psychiatrist at the Clinique Lyon Lumière, in Meyzieu, France. He holds degrees in neuroscience and in cognitive behavioral therapy, and combines his research with clinical experience in treating patients, including applications of meditation in a medical setting. Dr. Rosenfeld has played a major role in disseminating these applications in France, in particular with the publication of his book *Méditer c'est se soigner* (Meditating is self-care). He has practiced vipassana, Zen, and tai chi for a number of years.

Clifford Saron is an associate research scientist at the Center for Mind and Brain and the MIND Institute at the University of California, Davis. Saron has had a long-standing interest in the brain and behavioral effects of meditation practice. He has served as a faculty member at the Mind and Life Summer Research Institute and is currently a member of the Program and Research Council of the Mind and Life Institute. In the early 1990s—in collaboration with José Cabezón, Richard Davidson, Francisco Varela, B. Alan Wallace, and others, under the auspices of the Private Office of H.H. the Dalai Lama and the Mind and Life Institute—he was centrally involved in a field research project investigating Tibetan Buddhist mind training.

Saron is principal investigator of the Shamatha Project, working in collaboration with the Buddhist scholar B. Alan Wallace and a consortium of over thirty scientists and researchers at the University of California, Davis, and elsewhere. The project is the most comprehensive multimethod study to date of the effects of long-term intensive meditation practice. Saron's other primary research interest is investigating brain and behavioral correlates of sensory processing and multisensory integration in children on the autistic spectrum.

About the Editor

Andy Fraser is a London-based writer and editor with a special interest in meditation and Buddhism. After graduating from Cambridge University, he trained as a journalist and worked for the BBC, covering major sports events, including the 2004 Olympic Games in Athens. He has been practicing Tibetan Buddhism since 2002, and he regularly attends retreats at Lerab Ling in France, where the Meditation and Health conference took place. A prolific writer, Fraser is also the editor of *View, The Rigpa Journal,* an annual magazine on meditation and Tibetan Buddhism, which was founded in 2008.

Index